I0121849

even if i am.

even if i am.

an e-memoir

chasity glass

Shilhon House
9236 SW 40th Avenue
Portland, OR 97214

ISBN: 978-0-9856787-7-7
ISBN: 978-0-9856787-9-1 (e-book)
ISBN: 978-0-9856787-2-2 (multimedia e-book)

Cover and book design by Royal York Funston
www.ryarts.com

Printed in the United States of America
First Edition, 2012

for Anthony,
for my parents,
for my in-laws,
and for those
who've pedaled alongside me
on a bike ride…

preface

even if i am. is a true story.

It is both a book and an e-memoir because it is told in more than words. Pictures, audio interviews, music and web links in the multimedia e-book permit a truer and more personal telling. Apple's iPad supports this format today, and I highly recommend it for a complete experience. However, to share this story with a broader audience, it is also available as a printed book and standard e-book.

In the interest of privacy, some names, e-mail addresses, and other personal details have been replaced or removed. Otherwise, all e-mails, blog posts, audio clips, and photographs are actual and unaltered.

Over 12 million people are diagnosed with cancer each year.

This is the story of one... and the girl who loved him.

chapter one

inspiration information

PEOPLE ARE REALLY ROMANTIC ABOUT THE BEGINNING OF things. I'm reasoning this as my friend babbles on about how, for the first time, she is "experiencing love, instead of trying to figure it all out." She's saying she doesn't want to waste time on unnecessary boyfriends: "After all, I'm twenty-eight." She has a head full of doubt and a heart full of promise. "It feels as though I'm always thinking of him," she chirps, "and I just know somehow he's out there thinking of me." She then chatters on about fresh starts, clean slates and moving to Colorado for love.

I am still aware, distantly, of those late-twenties sentiments and world-of-possibility statements. I said them myself, about five years ago. I too thought that love—my own little bundle of doubt and promise—was neither A nor B. Love wasn't a right or left turn. Love was a continuum. It was the path to knowing everything would be all right. Knowing that "somehow he was out there thinking of me," and that I wasn't facing life alone. It's not that I believe in everlasting love anymore; I know better than to think in infinite terms now. Yet, if it weren't for some native sense of romance I wouldn't have done things like traveled to Australia on a whim or flown to Italy. I definitely wouldn't have volunteered to eat ten chocolate cupcakes in five minutes, helping raise money for cancer awareness. If it weren't for love I wouldn't have the words "even if i am" tattooed on my arm. I wouldn't have Anthony's last name.

"Oooh, good song..." My friend points to the ceiling as we listen to the music in the coffee shop we sit—"Hollow Talk" by Choir of Young Believers.

"Chas?" Her starry eyes shift as she asks, "Did you feel the same when you met Anthony?"

Her words rattle me.

The chorus sings, "Everything goes back to the beginning."

...

"My God, he's hot."

That was the first thing I ever said about him. *My God he's hot*, as if I was a fourteen year-old Valley Girl.

"Yeah, but someone THAT attractive has to have some major personal issues, right?" Emily's humor was always straight to the point. "I bet he's a total asshole."

She and I were standing at the copy machine. We just kept staring. It was hard not to. He was stunning. Tall and slender, fashionably messy dark hair complemented with a little stubble on his face. He wore a fuzzy black sweater over a white collared shirt and jeans… Even with a small moth hole in the shoulder, sexy. No question.

"I bet he sleeps with girls on first dates," Emily sneered.

"I bet he doesn't even go on first dates, just functions with one-nighters."

Surely he heard Emily and I snickering because he turned toward us. His smile was the last thing I expected.

"Oh, shit. Emily. QUICK! Copy something."

He looked down at his feet in embarrassment and returned to his conversation. He glanced back to see if we were still staring, sent another sexy half-smile in my direction.

"Okay, THAT smile is kind of hot."

"Yeah." I blushed, too. "I'd sleep with him on a first date."

…

I had just started working at Creative, the overtly trendy post-production house that now included a DVD department. My first assignment was to help drive some dramatic project revolving around Bette Davis and Joan Crawford.

"OHMYGOD!" I could hear Emily screech while running into my office, "You will NEVER guess who we have for an editor!"

Oh hell. "You've got to be kidding me. Out of fifteen editors…"

Emily was an excellent coordinator. Her dry wit complemented my sarcasm. Even as she updated me on the particulars of the project, she felt comparable to a cold beer on a hot day and a good long laugh. "Go downstairs and introduce yourself. When you get back, call me with the details. I'll put money down that he tries to sleep with you."

"Well then, I better introduce myself."

...

I'm not sure why the company was arranged on two floors, producers on the seventh, editors on the sixth. Space, I guess. Most took the elevator. I liked the stairs. Plus, the bathroom was on the way. I could fix my hair before the introduction.

I was apprehensive. Especially since I insulted him an hour ago. *Please God, tell me he didn't hear that.* I walked slowly until I stood at his door, hesitating as a noisy rock ballad escaped from behind it. I lifted my fist to knock, considered how I'd actually introduce myself if he had heard the insult. Our boss Kaethy turned the corner, headed toward me. I quickly knocked, appearing busy.

"Come in."

He turned from his computer and smiled broadly, easily persuading me to enter.

"HI, I'M CHAS," I yelled over the loud music.

He turned it down. "Ahhh, so you're the producer assigned to clean up this mess of a project. I'm Anthony."

He stood to shake my hand, stumbling around his desk and coffee table. A true gentleman. His excitable smile made me smile. Huge. And he smelled good. Damn good. I took a deep inhale, then realized I was still shaking his hand. Minutes passed, possibly days. *Silence. Awkward. Do I even know English? Words. Speak. Produce!* I immediately dropped his hand like a hot potato.

"Soooo, where are we at with the project now?" *Smooth. Chas, real smooth.* Then wiped my clammy palm on my jeans.

I was anxious, but our dialogue flowed as we discussed the Bette Davis and Joan Crawford assignment. Nerves had me chatting too casually, asking questions about previous careers, college. I even told Anthony about working at a gas station in high school, describing it as my favorite job, because I "liked the outfit, a striped shirt."

"Well," I said, cutting myself short, "I suppose I should get back to my desk. By now I'll have hundreds of e-mails to reply to."

"Hey, one more question before you go."

"Sure."

"Were you and Emily checking me out earlier today?" Again, with that sexy half-smile.

"Maybe?" I teased.

"I thought so."

I gave Anthony an awkward grin and quickly closed his office door behind me, practically ran out of there before he asked if I had insulted him too. On the commute back to my desk, I replayed our conversation in my mind. I wondered if he was really amused with my gas pumping abilities or just humoring me. Probably the latter. Asshole.

. . .

Back at my computer, I checked my e-mail. The inbox was overflowing, but I only noticed the most recent arrival.

From: le_samurai@yahoo.com
To: cturnquist@creative.com
Sent: Wednesday, February 16, 6:09 p.m.
Subject: inspiration

I just wanted to say "hi."
again.
in hopes to spark another conversation with you,
or inspiration in you,
or at least give us a continued recess
from our good friends bette & joan.

a.

I couldn't believe Anthony e-mailed. Emily was right. Total player.

From: cturnquist@creative.com
To: le_samurai@yahoo.com
Sent: Wednesday, February 16, 6:15 p.m.
Subject: Re: inspiration

don't you have work you should be doing
for a particular producer?

ok, let's see...
conversation filler for a continued recess.

since I've already given you some basics,
just moments ago.
time for something obscure.
I'm a huge Gene Kelly fan. (Obscure enough?)

For the first 16 years of life, I was quite positive I was going to be the next Gene Kelly, Ben Vereen, Gregory Hines, Sammy Davis or Bo Jangles. As a kid I wanted posters of all these tap dancers to line my bedroom wall... a bit geeky I know.

do I still tap?
ummmm...
I own tap shoes?

Chas

I called Emily directly after pushing "send." After all, she knew I was crushing on him. She'd be my ally. I couldn't tell any of my other friends. I knew they would judge, pry, poke and pick at the details. I didn't have to explain to Emily. She saw Anthony's smiles, and my blushing, grinning replies. "Heaven help you," she'd taunt. Sure, she could be brash and judgmental, but she believed in fairytale love. She was in love—a minister's daughter with a Jewish boyfriend. She believed love was a Woody Allen movie ending with a perfect kiss. She trusted wholly in love, said, "You'd be a FOOL to believe otherwise."

Besides, she was nosy and wanted to share in my work scandal.

"I waited for you to get back to your office, but you were in his edit bay FOREVER. Sooo, what happened?"

I described the clumsy handshake and his smile. Of course I dished the details of the conversations, his e-mail, and my response. We recapped the embarrassing copy machine incident, mocking our fear when Anthony turned to us. We burst out laughing.

"Okay, I'm home now. See you tomorrow."

As I hung up the phone I entered my apartment and was greeted by Gladys, quite possibly the ugliest dog in the world. "Hello, beautiful," I told her. She danced around, tapping her feet on the tiled kitchen floor, snorting and barking with excitement, when I heard a familiar voice behind me.

"I thought that was you." He kissed me with the same quick peck as he had done for the past five years, and once again my boyfriend asked me how my day was. I began to tell him as he went back to his computer and returned to his work. I'm not sure he ever really heard how my day was, but every night he asked. And every night I gave the bland, edited version of my day as he focused on his computer screen.

I'm not going to use his name in this story. I'll call him *Five Year*, which might seem heartless, but looking back, the relationship seems like such a long time ago that really, his name doesn't matter. In the scheme of things, that relationship is about the time I had invested in it, and not who I was dating. Anyway, I had a boyfriend, and a routine. A five-year routine I had grown comfortable and content with. A routine I labeled love. Maybe it wasn't fairytale love like Emily's; maybe we weren't riding off in the sunset bareback on a horse—but it was called love.

"What do you want for dinner?" I asked. *Whatever*, I silently mouthed his response as I stood at the fridge, hoping an answer would present itself. "How about breakfast for dinner?" I hollered across the apartment.

"Breakfast for dinner? You know I never like that. Let's just order Thai food."

And with that, another night of routine passed. Another night of work reports, computer screens, nighttime television dramas and halfhearted conversations. Some nights included slamming doors, yelling petty reasons why our relationship was flawed, or arguing compromises. The fights broke up the monotony.

even if i am.

From: le_samurai@yahoo.com
To: cturnquist@creative.com
Sent: Thursday, February 17, 12:53 p.m.
Subject: inspiration information

quite the colorful tapestry you are...

i suppose there is a day
when we have to take our posters down,
but it makes me wonder about yours...
what happened when you were 16?
that you stopped tapping.
...and when the heck
will i get to see you dance???

i played piano.
i'm trying not to make it sound trite
(most everyone took lessons as a child, right?)
but i played from first grade
until sometime around seventh grade
(see also: sometime around girls)

and although it was classical training,
it was always very solitary, very personal,
and a place to learn music, rhythm,
and most of all expression—

so
we'll hit the road:
i'll play piano,
you tap.
we'll rock the club circuit
and show the world something
they ain't never seen...

or maybe i'll just sit in my edit bay
and finish this damn bette and joan project

a.

p.s. please feel free to stop by anytime

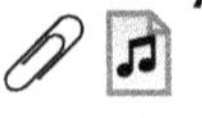
"Inspiration Information"
Shuggie Otis

From: cturnquist@creative.com
To: le_samurai@yahoo.com
Sent: Thursday, February 17, 1:16 p.m.
Subject: Re: inspiration information

kicking it old school
with a little Shuggie Otis attached...
nice touch.

even if i am.

Chas fact #2:
My father is a musician. He lives in the backwoods of Minnesota (by himself of course) and plays the blues. Sorta well known around town, and has been in a band since he was young. Bass. As a kid, I think he tried to teach me life lessons through a blues, jazz, or funk song...

If I just broke up with my boyfriend maybe a little John Lee Hooker, or failed some math test how about James Cotton, or maybe a bit depressed he'd throw in Robert Johnson and then tell me the story about the crossroads. (If you don't know the famed story, you should.)

If I was confused, worried or excited...
how about some Parliament-Funkadelic.

So although all kids took piano lessons, I took bass lessons. I played in a band throughout high school, and then stopped.

just like dance...
I stopped.
hmmmm.
not sure why,
I just did.
grew up I guess.

you should take piano lessons again.
I mean, you're gonna have to practice

if we start gigging right?

in the meantime
I better look like I'm working!
anymore Anthony fun facts?

Chas

After our morning meeting, my boss and a handful of co-workers were headed back to our desks when there Anthony was, walking toward us in the hall. I was so incredibly excited to see him. I mean, come on: model good-looking. Granted, we were only day two in our e-mail rapport, but I felt like I was in junior high. I wanted to jump up and down, grab someone's arm and point. "Ohmygod, thereheis, hessocute!" However, our boss was next to me. Co-workers, too. I was thrilled, pleased, charmed, overjoyed, and completely elated to see him, but I played it so cool that I hardly looked at him. I ignored his endearing hello as we passed. *Ohmygod.* I was right—just like junior high, and just as smooth.

From: le_samurai@yahoo.com
To: cturnquist@creative.com
Sent: Friday, February 18, 1:46 p.m.
Subject: game face

anthony fun facts…
nothing nearly as interesting

even if i am.

as a backwoods bluesman, the bass,
or parliament-funkadelic

i was raised by a single mom,
in the suburbs of washington DC,
with two adopted brothers—
(the three of us together are a sight)
and we raised each other
while my mother finished grad school
and began working at children's hospital
as a developmental psychologist for premature infants—
i can't quite explain what it was like
to have a psychologist for a mother,
but i can tell you,
i still smell it
in my every fiber—

i think i've always been a loner,
but usually feel better about it
when it is a choice
rather than the alternative—

my favorite color used to be orange,
when i was the only kid in the second grade
with a backpack of that color,
sometime later i decided green
was much more my style,
much more peaceful—

and am currently looking for the right color
to paint my room from the white it is now...

i live in a six-bedroom house with five others,
an accommodation i am surprised to admit
i have been in for four years—
it sounds absurd, but it is actually
quite nice, comforting, and quaint—

my quiet pleasure are my plants,
which i have picked up at various times
over the years, but water them all on saturdays—

i was born on january 23rd
and although it's cheesy,
my eyes always seem to find the clock at 1:23—
a number that always seems to find me...

this must be sent now
as i've been picking at it all morning—
you doin' okay today?
you seemed a little preoccupied when I passed you,
but maybe that's just your game face—
lord knows that's mine

a.

p.s. my favorite parliament song is "the goose"

even if i am.

From: cturnquist@creative.com

To: le_samurai@yahoo.com

Sent: Friday, February 18, 3:54 p.m.

Subject: Re: game face

yep, that's the game face.
crazy morning meeting,
but I am back to sane.
no, more like balanced.

two adopted bothers eh?
and just your mom?
how about dad?

Me, I'm an only child. I grew up with my mom in a trailer park. Sounds rather redneck on paper. My folks were just kids when they had me. Seventeen. They didn't have much time to raise a daughter—they were still sorting out their own lives. Matter of fact, they still are.

you, a loner?
you don't seem like the loner type.

my favorite color is red.
but I am rather fond of green and purple.
you should paint your room green.
it represents healing and relaxation.

a six bedroom house with five others!
that sounds rather tight.
not much room for privacy.
is it all guys? like a frat house?

I am rather fond of plants myself.

Chas fun fact #3:
I used to be a landscape designer,
and I water my patio full of plants
on wed nights.

born on July 20.
are we not giving out years for a reason?

okay, okay, the REAL question.
why haven't you asked me if I have a boyfriend yet?
or do you already know the answer?
or maybe it doesn't matter?

I anxiously await a response...

Chas

I should've been working, but instead I passed the time waiting for his e-mailed reply listening to Shuggie Otis's "Inspiration Information" every three minutes. Over and over. Like a schoolgirl, I'd sing, "You making me happier, now I am snappier, while I'm with you." Between each lyric, I checked my inbox to see if he replied.

"You making me happier..."

Nope.

"Now I am snappier..."

Still no.

"While I'm with you..."

Repeat song. Twelve more times.

"You making..."

Finally!

From: le_samurai@yahoo.com
To: cturnquist@creative.com
Sent: Friday, February 18, 5:51 p.m.
Subject: words worth

music was made to suit our moments,
and it is part of life's game
to rediscover the music that fits
the moments we are living—

i hope this song finds you that way.

although your game face was a bit severe—
i too can be serious at times,
but know that there is another side to that coin—
a side that is goofy, playful,
and sometimes just plain retarded.

inspiration information

the story of my daddy is a long one,
and one i will tell you another time—
instead, i will address
the juicier questions you brought up...

i heard (this sounds so stupid)
that you have a boyfriend—
but didn't feel like it entered
into the equation of coming to understand
who you are—not yet, anyway.

i don't want to paint your picture
in the shadow of your relationship—
instead i would rather come to understand you,
all of your "facts" and idiosyncrasies
before learning how you relate
to someone else—

did i feel like i was in seventh grade
when i saw you this morning in the hallway?
certainly.

after sending you my e-mail,
did i check every five minutes
to see if you had written back?
absolutely.

even if i am.

do i feel guilty for geeking out
even though you have a boyfriend?
not at all.

reading your words
and writing my own
is a simple, beautiful pleasure
and one that defies circumstances—

besides, there is so much left to write
before we get to those chapters,
it would seem a shame to jump ahead...

a.

p.s. write back soon

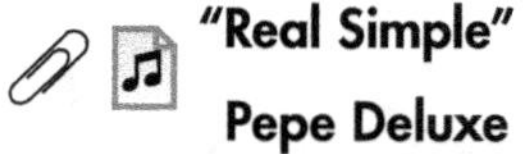

"Real Simple"
Pepe Deluxe

That night the melody kept my speed as the chorus drove me home. Home to a three-day weekend. Home to my routine. Home to Five Year.

Keeping it real simple
Making me feel so simple
Being close you know
If you're trying to make me

Feel uneasy
You're doing it right baby.

Knowing my pleasure in reading his e-mails, and writing my own, I wondered if we could "keep it simple." I wondered why he attached this particular song. Dissected the lyrics. Overanalyzed the e-mails. Wondering why his words were written like song lyrics themselves, and how strange it was that my own writing fell into his rhythm so quickly. Believing in things like chance and fate. Thinking about our conversations, driving home in a daydream. Letting the song mark the moment. Only three days since I saw him at the copy machine. Three days and I was falling. I had a head full of doubt and a heart full of promise. Then again, I'm *really* romantic about the beginning of things.

chapter two

real simple

When you're in a long-term relationship and work a nine-to-five job, three-day weekends are the rage. You get to catch up on fun tasks like grocery shopping and laundry. As I strolled through an overcrowded Trader Joe's with my boyfriend, this weekend was no exception.

Grocery shopping meant visits to three different stores so we could buy the brand names Five Year preferred. We weren't the kind of couple that held hands while perusing the shelves. We came in to buy and get out. Five Year would tackle the frozen foods while I hit the dairy section. We were a disciplined grocery shopping team with years of practice.

"Hey, I think we're out of toothpaste," I yelled down aisle three.

He agreed as he headed toward the pasta sauce. "They don't carry Colgate, though," he shouted back.

"I'll check to see what they have?"

As I scanned the limited Trader Joe's selection of toothpaste, I discovered a brand named Tom's of Maine. *Hmm. I wonder if this is any good.* I read the ingredients on the back of the box, then screwed open the cap to smell. It didn't smell Colgate fresh, but I figured we could try something different. It's natural, I thought. He might go for that. I threw it in the cart and moved on to the bread aisle.

As we stood in the checkout line unloading the cart, Five Year noticed the Tom's of Maine and set it aside.

"I like the taste of Colgate," he confirmed.

"Can't we try something new?"

"You can if you want, but I'm still gonna get Colgate at the other store."

Provoked, I put the toothpaste back on the conveyer belt.

...

As I got ready for bed that night, I saw the Tom's of Maine sitting next to the Colgate. I couldn't wait to use it. I opened the cap and squeezed the usual amount onto my toothbrush and started brushing. Up, down, right, left. Rinse. Repeat. WOW! This was the freshest tasting toothpaste I had ever experienced. It burned my gums, but in an "I'm-killing-bacteria-and-bad-breath" kind of way. As I scrubbed my teeth, I wondered why I hadn't used this before. No seriously though. It's better for you, it's natural, and it's so incredibly fresh tasting.

"Doesn't that stuff taste horrible? Isn't Colgate better?" Five Year asked, as he passed the bathroom.

Is Colgate better? Do I even like Colgate? Have I settled on a type of toothpaste? I started thinking back to the kinds of toothpaste I had used in previous relationships. I backtracked to my childhood, when my parents bought the toothpaste. I remember it being three different colors swirled together. I even remember the time when we ran out, and my mother made me brush my teeth with baking soda and water. Definitely memorable. But Colgate? When did I decide I preferred Colgate? I couldn't mark a definitive time. Had I really settled on a toothpaste for him? Five Year was set in his ways. Granted he was twelve years older and, as he explained throughout our relationship, "I've had more time to figure out what I like." This toothpaste incident was the perfect example. He was certainly not going to try something different. Why did I think he would? He knew what he preferred. These battles I had lost many times before. Why should toothpaste be any different? *Am I so dependent that I can't pick out my own toothpaste? Am I overreacting? It's just toothpaste, right?*

Confused, I crawled into bed and turned off the light. "I'm going to sleep now," I yelled toward our living room. "Come tuck me in."

even if i am.

...

Since high school I've had one relationship after another. It didn't help that I reversed my formative years; I maximized promiscuity in high school, and then suffered teen angst in my college dropout years. All the other girls were happily moving forward, striving towards careers in anthropology, business, and communications; seeking spouses and white picket fences. I cranked up the harsh heartbreak of Sarah McLachlan while they graduated with business degrees or married high school sweethearts. I contemplated my adolescence while exacerbating my despair by camouflaging my individuality in relationships.

I would chase men like other girls declared majors, each one giving me something to believe in, something to strive towards, and something to graduate with. Once in love, I'd disappear. I'd give up my being to the comfort of being in someone's arms—everything I had, everything I was. Self-identity seemed unnecessary as I struggled to understand love.

Of course after months of dating, I'd eventually blame and criticize my partner for not being "good enough." I'd find reasons to get out. He's too ugly, too romantic, too nice, too pathetic, too energetic, too old, too young, too close, too different. Did he always chew with his mouth open? I'd blame the disgusting sound of him chewing, stating, "I could never stay in *that* relationship," then seamlessly pick a different major with barely a summer's break. I was in a rut, a big, fat rut, and I didn't know how to get out of it.

chapter three

lovely day

From: le_samurai@yahoo.com
To: cturnquist@creative.com
Sent: Monday, February 21, 8:44 a.m.
Subject: so cool

it feels good to write to you now,
from the peace and quiet of my house
instead of the distractions and deadlines of work—

oh, the house... right:
of the six people here, four are men, two are women—
all young professionals in different fields.
except for jay—he is one of my closest friends,
works in the industry as a DP/Videographer,
and i went to Peru with him last month
to celebrate my 30th birthday.

even if i am.

not including my year of birth in the other e-mail
was completely unintentional—
turning 30 is another topic
we should discuss at some point—
fascinating stuff.

putting my personal life on the table:

i recently came to the end of a flawed,
tumultuous, soap-operatic relationship
that over the course of four months
managed to reach incredible heights
before crashing to an unexpected
but predictable end...
cryptic, i know.
details await.
and yes, i realize we have a backlog of topics,
and am eager for us to find a venue
to sit down and talk about
all the topics that are waiting for words...

if you're not insane with work,
let's try to have lunch, take a walk for coffee,
if you're feeling very brave, let's have dinner
and give each other an opportunity to really speak

a.

P.S. Attached is a photo on Machu Picchu from my birthday.

From: cturnquist@creative.com
To: le_samurai@yahoo.com
Sent: Tuesday, February 22, 11:34 a.m.
Subject: Re: so cool

ahh, the relationship:
the rumor mill has caught up with you too...
though, I think we might be getting our information
from a similar source.
starts with an E,
ends with a Y
and has mil in between?

I knew about your messy breakup.
no details really,
just that you broke up,
got hurt,
in recovery...

that and I've heard you're a nice guy.
not the asshole I figured you to be when we first met.
a good conversation for later maybe?

dinner eh?
honestly as much as I would love to take you up on the offer,
I am not sure I'd be comfortable with dinner...

even if i am.

at least not yet.

plus I think you and I alone in a room
(outside of work) spells t-r-o-u-b-l-e...
especially because you think I'm beautiful.

lunch, coffee, walks, all sound great!

I have to let you know that my hesitation is not only because I have a boyfriend, but because my boyfriend is a client here at work. Makes me a little more cautious of my actions...

am I scaring you off yet?
not my intention.

sorry for this rather problematic e-mail.
guess I should get back to this thing called producing...
maybe later I'll stop by for a visit.
I could use a smile.

...

Anthony was absolutely addicting. I got high with every e-mail, song or chance run-in. Confession: I used the sixth floor bathroom because it was next to his office. Only a wall separated us. Pathetic, right? I was infatuated, practically obsessed. Love makes me do stupid things.

...

From: le_samurai@yahoo.com
To: cturnquist@creative.com
Sent: Tuesday, February 22, 1:49 p.m.
Subject: for your eyes only

yes, your situation upstairs
sounds increasingly complex,
potentially problematic,
and ultimately shitty—

so come downstairs for a visit,
and we'll close the door
on peering eyes, misperceptions,
and unnecessary explanations—

if we can't have dinner,
can I walk you to your car tonight?

From: cturnquist@creative.com
To: le_samurai@yahoo.com
Sent: Tuesday, February 22, 3:42 p.m.
Subject: Re: for your eyes only

yes, I'd like that.

It felt like junior-high meeting at our lockers. I ran down to Anthony's office, stopped just before I could see him standing there, one foot leaning against the wall, nervously waiting. We clumsily smiled at one another.

Nerves had me chatty again as I rambled on about my current work project. He interrupted, "I like you." Just like that. A simple sentence.

"I know you do," thinking it was flirty banter.

"No, seriously."

"You mean like, like?" Clearly, still in junior high mode.

He nodded.

I didn't know how to respond.

"I didn't mean to just throw that at you," he said, "but I needed to say it."

"Why?"

"Because, I like you, and… I don't know. You standing here, talking, I just… needed to tell you, to see if you felt the same way, or if it's something I'm creating."

"I don't know what to say."

"Say what you feel."

I searched for words, as the muscles in my neck tensed. "Honestly, I'm confused. I've been in a relationship for five years and in those five years… I've never felt this excited to stand next to someone." Long pause. "Is that what you wanted to hear?"

He smiled. "Yeah, kind of."

"But why?" I was annoyed. I was in a relationship. He knew that. "I still have a boyfriend. Plus, you just got out of this same triangle situation, and I'm not wanting to be your new challenge." I didn't think. Just spoke. It was a rumor that he was in a triangle situation. I was mad, so I took a jab.

"Really, is that what you think this is to me? A challenge?"

"I don't know." I knew that sentence would piss him off.

"I wasn't expecting these feelings, but here they are, and I just needed you to know. Since the moment I saw you, I've had a crush on you."

"And I have one on you. Now what?"

"I don't know." He lingered. "My guess is you drive home?"

I was angry. At what, I don't even know. Maybe mad at myself for feeling those things. Guilty for telling him those things. I just stood there, quiet. I didn't know what to say. Nor did he. Two adults with junior high crushes. I thought it couldn't get more awkward until he smiled devilishly.

"Or we could drive to Mexico and elope?"

That damn smile got me every time. Every. Single. Time.

...

From: le_samurai@yahoo.com

To: cturnquist@creative.com

Sent: Tuesday, February 22, 11:08 p.m.

Subject: music for your daddy

11 p.m., and i just got home.

(have a feeling my drive and your drive were very similar.)

replaying our moments again,

even if i am.

wondering why i was so retarded—
and thinking that if we were seventh graders in the hallway,
we must have regressed a few years
as we stood by your car—

i wonder if your dad's music has answers
for all the questions we have now...

"the goose" has a special place in my heart,
and a story that i will tell you one day
(along with all the rest of the stories).
but this song, is one that goes way back (yonder)
and one that i could hear
when you told me about your daddy,
the backwoods, and the bass.

i hope you come to see me again,
even though our project is finished,
finding time between your schedule and mine
to sit in my office and share a smile at least—
and i hope we start to find our way
toward that rare level of comfort and understanding
that i know we are capable of...

do you think I can walk you to your car again?

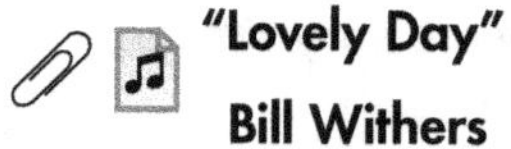

chapter four

ghost of things to come

TWENTY-SOMETHING LOVE IS ABSURD. THAT RUSH AND fluster over little things, like why he hadn't e-mailed that day. Why I hadn't heard from him all afternoon. Girls are simple: We just need a text or an e-mail or a phone call, a little something to remind us that the people we love are out there, thinking of us. Otherwise we stress. We create obscene circumstances of what went wrong.

I wondered if I should call Anthony or go down to his office, or maybe I should write another e-mail. I wondered if he was mad at me for something. I had insecurities of what I said, did, wore. All because I didn't get a morning e-mail.

Looking back it seems so foolish, all this self doubt, when it was the big events I should've been fretting over—the big mythological themes of life and death, of love and limited time. That's what matters, I know that now. Five years later, I try explaining it to my friends, though most don't understand. The only person who would understand is... Well, you, Anthony.

...

From: le_samurai@yahoo.com
To: cturnquist@creative.com
Sent: Thursday, February 24, 5:30 p.m.
Subject: life cycle

feeling a little out of sorts,
for a variety of reasons:
family is on the verge of a civil war,
i don't feel very good,
a broken love is calling for seconds,
and then of course, there's you.

instinct dives into work
and doesn't look back,
second guess looks back,
stupidity turns,
and before long
i'm in it.

in school,
math was the easiest topic—
formulas and equations,
rules and absolutes.

ghost of things to come

in life,
that's far from the case.
and yet, my mind searches
for the simple addition and resulting sum,
the clean division with no remainder—
it just isn't there

and that sucks.

my family is coming apart at the seams,
and i want more than anything
to find the magical words
that make everyone smile again,
and forgive each other—

but the fact that i am discovering
and slowly coming to terms with,
is that my family has never been
as close as i thought they were—
my mother and her siblings
have a beef that goes back fifty years...
fifty years!
that's fucking insane!

i have made my own way into the arena.
weapons are drawn, but is this my fight?

even if i am.

my health is questionable these days.
i have a stomach ache that won't go away.
chalk it up to stress, i guess.

then there's broken love,
calling for seconds
in the shadow of her husband
and that's a whole other story—
a story that refuses to end
but needs to.

and finally you,
my beautiful friend:
this breath that blows in
and escapes just before i can take it in,
a curious cat that comes close
but always stays just out of reach,
an answer that leaves more questions.

life goes in cycles.
usually when one cycle
reaches a boiling/turning point—

i think i'm there
with a stomach ache.

From: cturnquist@creative.com
To: le_samurai@yahoo.com
Sent: Thursday, February 24, 6:14 p.m.
Subject: the rotation of life

I myself can surely relate to the struggles of family ties,
being in the middle of a battle I was never a part of.
not to mention I was never very good at picking a side,
hence living as many miles away from family as possible.
hence visiting them on my terms, when I need.

the only way I make it through...
is remembering that their actions
don't reflect mine.

some battles are lost standing on the sidelines.

I, on the other hand, am weakest in math.
I question matter-of-fact formulas,
and I definitely don't live for rules and absolutes...
just possibilities.

it is within those "remainders"
from our "clean division"
that keeps life in flux and makes it interesting.

as for a love calling for seconds...
only you know what's best.

even if i am.

only you can answer those feelings,
remember those pasts,
embrace those emotions.

if you think going back to a past relationship
would in any way change this...
it doesn't.
it couldn't.

and although there is a breath
that escapes before you take it in
it's consistent and genuinely...
a possibility.

so. smile. I am.

maybe I can rub your tummy to make it feel better?

From: le_samurai@yahoo.com
To: cturnquist@creative.com
Sent: Thursday, February 24, 6:23 p.m.
Subject: Re: the rotation of life

thank you.
i am smiling now
oh. you rubbing my tummy sounds lovely.

I didn't want to pry. It was none of my business. I thought maybe I could be an ear, a friend. A connection to look forward to at the end of the day. I'd be perky and fun (instead of my sarcastic self) to get Anthony's mind off of heavy thoughts.

When he wasn't waiting for me outside his office door, it stung a little. Instead I knocked and asked if he was ready, waited for him to collect his belongings. He didn't say a word, just nodded yes. No witty banter, no teasing, he said nothing as we headed to our cars. I strolled alongside as close as I could, leaning on his arm. I wanted to cheer him up somehow, nudged him with my head to get a response. Like a kitten circling his feet, waiting to be touched. I practically meowed. When we got to my car, he merely said, "Goodnight."

There was no walking back and forth, no prolonged goodbye. We parked next to each other. I didn't know what to do, so I climbed into his truck, closed the door and stared straight ahead at the cement wall of the parking structure. It was dark, and few cars remained in the garage. I can't say I wasn't nervous when he climbed in the driver's seat. Unsteady, he turned on his iPod, as quiet music began to fill the space.

"Your tummy feeling better?" I purred. Never thinking this would become an often-asked question.

"It will be after you rub it."

There was a deep worry in his voice. He reached for my hand, slowly touching my knuckles with the tip of his finger. The affection sent shivers through every part of me. My hand reached for his.

Our fingers expressed the passion our bodies could not, speaking the fervor our words did not. He and I said nothing, expressing everything in our caresses. Our hands intertwined, squeezed, tangled and fondled. Clasped so tight we watched them move to the rhythm of the music as the car radio sang to us, for us. We simply held hands.

What felt like minutes soon became an hour. I didn't want it to end. Even now the thought of it sends shivers. (And babe, I'd hold your hand every damn time if it would've helped any tummy aches go away.)

"I should probably go." I was mostly trying to convince myself, though.

Hesitating, Anthony opened my palm and drew a heart in the center of it. "Take this with you. Be careful. It's fragile," Then he closed my hand.

I got out of the car with my hand still closed, as he drove away. I didn't want him to leave. I wanted him to turn around, pick me up and take me out of my routine. Drive to Mexico.

ghost of things to come

...

From: le_samurai@yahoo.com
To: cturnquist@creative.com
Sent: Friday, February 25, 10:01 a.m.
Subject: moments

thank you for last night.
it felt very much overdue
to sit down with you,
and share a moment
we have only alluded to...

attached is a song that was playing

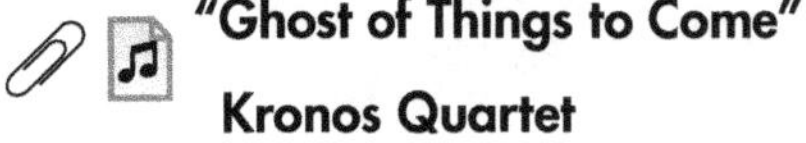

I didn't respond to Anthony's e-mail all day. I avoided the sixth floor. I shunned overwhelming feelings of pleasure from the night before. I chastised myself: I HAVE A BOYFRIEND. I wrote it down on a sticky note and stuck it to my computer screen as a reminder to not e-mail. I somehow avoided him for most of the day. When we ran into each other in the lunchroom, I blamed work for my distance. "I am SOOO busy today, sorry." It wasn't a complete lie.

I snuck out of the office without saying goodnight, and headed home for the weekend.

chapter five

la cienega just smiled

"ARE YOU TRYING TO PICK A FIGHT?" FIVE YEAR YELLED.

"No," I said, using my indoor voice.

"Then why are you bringing this up again?" Still yelling. "Don't we have enough pressure on our relationship? Plus, you just started a new job. Things need to be settled before we start thinking about marriage." He stormed out of the room.

"But it's been five years." I followed him. "We've lived together for four? How *settled* does it need to be?"

"When our relationship is perfect, maybe then," he snapped. "Why can't it just stay the way it is? Next you're going to ask me if I want kids, and you already know that answer. I told you from the beginning of our relationship that I don't want kids. Why are you picking a fight?"

"I'm not. I just asked you if we'll ever get married. You're the asshole yelling."

"We are done with this conversation." He slammed the door behind him.

...

From: cturnquist@creative.com
To: le_samurai@yahoo.com
Sent: Monday, February 28, 6:02 p.m.
Subject: another e-mail

here is my e-mail,
an e-mail I wrote today...
each time I came to my desk,
I'd type a sentence more.

I needed a chance to really think
about our moments together,
and so I spent the entire weekend
consumed by thoughts of you...
potentials.
possibilities.
complications.

I realized that since "this" started
I have been so caught up in my own emotions and confusions
that I never factored in yours.
I had heard you were in a messy triangle situation
but I assumed your heart

to be secure, not fragile.

so here is where I stand...

you deserve
first dates,
first kisses,
and unexpected love,
without sneaking around
and worrying about boyfriends or husbands...

Plus I don't want you to be a home-wrecker, and given where my relationship stands with my boyfriend, "this" would be just another triangle situation. Another equation that you are all too familiar with. I told you in the beginning that I am not engaged, but if he asked me tomorrow, my answer would be yes. With that said, my relationship for the past few months (long before you) has been difficult and trying. We are at a crossroads where we either commit or move on. As each day passes, my ideas for the future, for marriage and children, change, making my relationship with my boyfriend strenuous.

I am far too intrigued by our conversations,
far too emotionally involved,
and inundated with feelings of infatuations,
that I do not want to be,
nor do I want you to be,
a rebound or an affair...

even if i am.

I'd much rather
just be your friend.

I'll be the first to admit that sexual tensions can get the best of a situation, and being alone in a room with you I imagine rather difficult. But, I respect our relationship thus far, and I don't want that to change. I am attracted to you. However, we need to sort out our lives, loves and futures without worrying or questioning "this."

so, as often as I think about you
or you of me...
let's get to know each other, let's flirt, let's be friends,
but let's sort out other things
before anything else.
deal?

From: le_samurai@yahoo.com
To: cturnquist@creative.com
Sent: Monday, February 28, 6:50 p.m.
Subject: Re: another e-mail

it had been a strange day:
to see you for a moment, aloof and indifferent—
a far cry from the person i have come to know.

your e-mail arrived

la cienega just smiled

and was a welcome change:
honest and open,
brave and articulate—
thank you for that.

there are many levels on which we interact,
and i am fascinated by all of them—
however, although they intersect,
they are also independent, and i sincerely believe
we can become friends, healthy friends,
not hiding an obvious attraction,
but not acting on it—

i agree with you in that the circumstances
are way too much (like, soap-operatic much)
and it is no small relief to sidestep
the potential complications,
to explore each other's safer sides,
and to let our friendship blossom
out in the open and in the light,
instead of the dark closet of secrets—

you are amazing.
brilliant and beautiful—
and i am thankful
for your every word
and every minute.

even if i am.

"La Cienega Just Smiled"
Ryan Adams

We would stand by this agreement for the next five months. I never wanted to hurt Five Year. That was never my intention. I honestly believed I wasn't cheating. Looking back it's totally stupid. I know. I had crossed the line, maybe not physically but surely emotionally. Something in me changed subtly, like the moment the tide turns. Five years held so much weight. I hadn't committed to five years of anything in my life—the closest was saxophone lessons in middle school and that only lasted two years. When I imagined my old age, and tried to picture myself on the porch swing with someone, that person wasn't Five Year—truthfully, he never was. I never imagined us growing old together.

The song "La Cienega Just Smiled" held the pain of a breakup. The music and lyrics were absolutely crushing. Why? Because it was Anthony sitting next to me on that imagined porch swing. I knew it from the moment I met him. I was just too scared to admit that I felt this way about him, and Ryan Adams seemed to know it.

chapter six

flying high

"Thanks for coming to lunch. It was nice to see what color your eyes are."

"And what color are they?" Playfully turning my back.

Anthony spun me closer by a belt loop, encouraged by my tease. "Green, like mine." We were still giggling as we entered the office, his finger hooked in my loop.

"Hey Chas, where were you? We have a production meeting in ten minutes—" Emily turned around in my chair, where she was waiting. "OHHH," she said, as if surprised, "that's where you were. Hi, Anthony."

He responded with an awkward wave. Embarrassed, we said nothing, separated, and then parted ways.

"So?" Emily blurted.

"What?" I rolled my eyes at her.

even if i am.

...

From: le_samurai@yahoo.com
To: cturnquist@creative.com
Sent: Tuesday, March 1, 4:07 p.m.
Subject: the light of day

well, the light of day agrees with you...

if i ever get out for lunch,
we will have to do that again
without interruptions and uncomfortable goodbyes.
(our visits never seem long enough.)

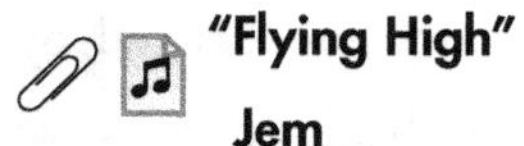

But I'm flying so high
High off the ground
When you're around
And I can feel your high
Rocking me inside
It's too much to hide

I know, oh yes
I know that we can't
Be together
But, I just like to dream

flying high

From: chasityrae@gmail.com
To: le_samurai@yahoo.com
Sent: Monday, March 1, 1:09 p.m.
Subject: the songs you send

last night
this weekend
every day

I fight with the idea
of seeing you.

I think about the consequences,
the repercussions.
and I don't care
if it means a moment
with you.

it's a struggle
to push feelings aside
to be rational

a battle I am losing…
I adore you.

the way you smile at me with green eyes
the way you grab my belt loop to pull me closer

even if i am.

your words
your thoughts
your e-mails,
and the songs you send...

I adore.

...

I did it. I confessed everything to Emily. I needed to tell someone. I admitted I was flirting at obnoxious levels, that I had crossed the friendship line but always tiptoed back to the safe side. I played her some of the songs he sent, like "Flying High." I told her about the dozens of e-mails sent in less than a month, never losing contact. I told her I knew about Anthony's current fling with a roommate, and of his rowdy nights with his best friend Jay. That he knew about my relationship with Five Year. I told her there was a sense of relief in getting to know Anthony without the weight of attachments. How we'd laugh too long. Sneak out for lunch. Give lingering goodbye hugs. I told her I couldn't get enough. I even confessed the secret conversations in the stairwell. I did. I told her everything.

"I love it!" Emily said, laughing and shaking her head. She wasn't surprised. She told me about how she too looked for that right person, trying to find a guy who was fun and sexy and funny. She confirmed those restless feelings of standing in that nowhere place, trying to find someone to love, someone to hold on to—and she found him. It was good to share those experiences with her. It's what brought us together as friends, because at that point in our lives we were experiencing the same feelings and emotions, the same sense of searching. Love in your twenties can be a confusing thing. It holds much more weight because you don't want to waste time or play games. You want to approach love with absolute faith.

Her truth was reassuring, and her delight, completely contagious.

chapter seven

don't stop

From: le_samurai@yahoo.com
To: chasityrae@gmail.com
Sent: Wednesday, March 2, 2:47 p.m.
Subject: good morning?

a strange mood for a strange day...
but i also think i'm feeling more
comfortable with you as a person,
and consequently am more
open/brave/inappropriate...

perhaps because we've ruled out
something happening between us,
it allows us to feel more comfortable
with flirting to obnoxious levels...
for example:

even if i am.

some of my favorite things in the world
are sex, spooning, and napping—
but done in perfect tandem with each other,
then, well, that's a lovely way
to spend a weekend afternoon—

but i wonder,
you seem so driven and intense—
i wonder how well you relax,
how good you are at lazy sundays,
and how much you enjoy
the things i enjoy...

the "brazilian girls" are playing sunday
at the knitting factory
and also tuesday at the temple bar—
me and jay do our best groupie impressions
and try to see them whenever they come to town...
might even go to both shows.

important note:
the name is not exactly accurate,
as there is only one girl in the band,
and she's from spain, italy, or something...

so i've attached another song,
and you really ought to be careful
with this one, cause it fuckin' thumps!

(and it's kinda sexy too...)

hmm.
this is me
slowly stepping back
behind the line.

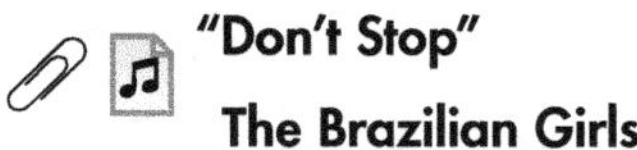

From: chasityrae@gmail.com
To: le_samurai@yahoo.com
Sent: Wednesday, March 2, 3:34 p.m.
Subject: Re: good morning?

well then.
ehum (clearing throat).
good thing I switched to my "private" e-mail address.

although I too like to spend a weekend afternoon
with sex, spooning and of course naps...
I can assure you our sexual appetites differ.

I can be intense
quite frisky
and surely hungry.

and this is beyond obnoxious flirting.

even if i am.

especially with a song like that.

From: le_samurai@yahoo.com

To: chasityrae@gmail.com

Sent: Wednesday, March 2, 3:45 p.m.

Subject: Re: good morning?

when was the last time you had sex?

From: chasityrae@gmail.com

To: le_samurai@yahoo.com

Sent: Wednesday, March 2, 4:01 p.m.

Subject: Re: good morning?

knowing your answer is probably last night...

remember I do have a steady boyfriend...
of five years.
which is sorta like being married.
so sex is less of a need.
more of a want.

not to mention,
my bedroom habits, and my last time
is really none of your business
since we ruled out our relationship
ever reaching this point.

monday.

Neither of us could control what was happening, in particular our physical attraction. I wanted to devour Anthony, kiss him, cuddle him—hell, even hugging him was satisfying. He was sexy, and talking about sex—talking about anything at this point was, well, sexy. I teetered from practical to improbable. I wasn't a cheater. *My God he's hot.* I lost myself in my attraction to him. The push and pull from lust to guilt had me spinning.

...

From: le_samurai@yahoo.com
To: chasityrae@gmail.com
Sent: Thursday, March 3, 9:31 a.m.
Subject: new day

a new day
new e-mail.

it would have been nice to see you,
to follow up all the written words
with a physical presence, and a smile—

but honestly, it did become frustrating
to think about you, visualize you
in all of your uninhibited beauty,

even if i am.

loving, being loved, and being free...
it is hard to smell the aroma
but not taste the dish...

and yes.
i am hungry.

but you were right,
in that sex does mean
different things to you and i—
the superficial appeal
does not deafen my ears
the way it once did,
but the loving i miss
and the loving i want
comes from as much of an emotional place
as it does a physical one—

the emotions we feel
with the one we are with,
elevates us into another dimension—

sheesh!
hot shit for first thing
in the morning

don't stop

From: chasityrae@gmail.com

To: le_samurai@yahoo.com

Sent: Thursday, March 3, 10:32 a.m.

Subject: Re: new day

you my friend, are a helpless romantic.
your ideas of love and intimacy are endearing.
you really need a girlfriend to adore!

I too prefer to have an emotional
as well as physical connection with someone.
to love. to be loved.

the only difference is...
I can keep them separate.
I can enjoy each one,
physical, emotional,
on separate levels.
to me they don't go hand in hand
but compliment each other,
whereas some need one to have the other.

I too agree that yesterday's conversation
may have been a little frustrating,
but I look for the possibilities...
and anxiously wait meals ahead.

even if i am.

From: le_samurai@yahoo.com
To: chasityrae@gmail.com
Sent: Thursday, March 3, 12:41 p.m.
Subject: Re: new day

i have been in love before,
beautiful, dizzy, inspired love—
and these days, anything less
seems like a waste of time.

too often in past relationships
i have felt the guilt and sadness
of an unbalanced relationship—
when one is loved more than they love...

my brother once told me
that all relationships
fall into that category,
and its just a matter
of what side of it you want to be on...
my mother told me once
that the side you're on oscillates with time...
christ. this is making my head hurt—

anyway,
last time i had sex was friday—
and it was sweet, safe, and comfortable...
not quite the adjectives i like.

you just came in, to give me a hug
and now i'm all thrown off...

...

I didn't even knock, I walked right in. Closed the door behind me.

"I'm a girl and that's what girls do. Sometimes we're aggressive and sometime we want to cuddle. And sometimes we sleep with men we don't love. We overanalyze things and sometimes we don't know what we want. At least, I don't know what I want. I get moody sometimes. I'm a girl. And I'm sorry if our e-mails felt feisty yesterday. Sometimes I get like that. You're just gonna have to deal with it." I opened my arms, and motioned my fingers inward. "Now give me a hug."

I talk too much when I'm nervous and sometimes I have this high-pitched, pouty whine. I'm a girl and that's what girls do. We whine.

chapter eight

breathe me

In between bites of pasta, Five Year continued, "I know we've been fighting a lot, especially the past few months. I know that you're trying to rediscover yourself, playing guitar and writing more..." He chewed, stammered on. "Hell, I remember being in my late twenties and needing to find my own again, too. I just hope this search doesn't affect our relationship. I want you to know that I love you, and I am completely content."

I shuddered at the word *content* but acknowledged his sincerity with a brief smile.

He didn't notice my cringe. "I'd hate for things to get more complicated between us. We seem to be fighting all the time. Even more since you've been rediscovering yourself. I do want you to enjoy those things again. I want to enjoy them with you. I'm just scared of losing you. I love you."

"I love you too."

I didn't know what else to say.

even if i am.

. . .

From: chasityrae@gmail.com
To: le_samurai@yahoo.com
Sent: Monday, March 28, 10:46 a.m.
Subject: hurt...

this e-mail is certainly NOT meant to hurt you,
but it will bring you no comfort or pleasure.

it is me simply being as honest as I can
with you
with myself.

I am crazy about you—
there is no denying that.
plus I think I tell you in every damn e-mail.

but it is becoming
much more than that.
feelings I can't control,
we can't control
feelings of love, yes, love
of passion.
of obsession.

feelings that scare me.
I hardly know you.

but am terrified by our likeness.

and throughout these feelings
I HAVE A BOYFRIEND!
a sweet and caring boyfriend.
who might not make my skin crawl with hunger.
who might not have the poetry of life,
and the passion of love in his fingertips,

but he is mine.
and I do love him.
and he loves me...
I am not sure I am ready to leave.
I am not sure I am strong enough.

you deserve to be loved.
and loved fully.

I CANNOT offer that.
I wish I could
but I cannot.

so I am asking you again.
I am hurting.

so before I hurt you,
as much if not more
than I am hurting myself...

even if i am.

walk away.
please.
I care too much about you.

today...
let's talk, get coffee, question...
then take a little time to sort out our lives?

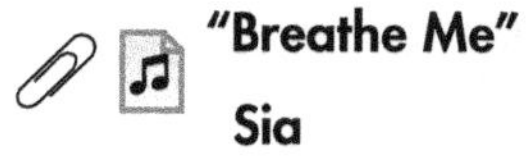
"Breathe Me"
Sia

We hadn't talked all day. My e-mail sat with no reply. I figured Anthony was upset when his voice on the phone asked me to meet him in the stairwell "right now." He hung up before I had the chance to respond. I was apprehensive. I walked slowly as I imagined him pacing, waiting, angry.

His watery eyes welcomed mine, soft and anxious. It caught me off guard when I opened the stairwell door and saw him on the top step. I dragged my feet as I climbed each stair. Charged with courage, he met me halfway on the staircase, then clutched my waist. Before I could say a word, he pressed my body against the wall to meet his. It all happened so fast. I felt his weight against mine and caught my breath. Eyes wide open, he placed his lips gently on my cheek, and then stopped as we both exhaled in one big breath. He knew what I was going to say before I said it.

We held our faces close, intimately rubbing cheeks, nuzzling noses, lips, ears, eyelashes, purely breathing each other in. Inhale. Exhale. Bodies pressed as close as clothes allowed.

We never kissed. We merely absorbed one another's breathing. Feeling only what we wanted to feel. Repeating smiles. The rest of the world didn't matter.

"Does this help sort things out?" His whisper kissed my cheek.

chapter nine

waiting for my real life to begin

From: le_samurai@yahoo.com

To: chasityrae@gmail.com

Sent: Thursday, April 14, 11:06 a.m.

Subject: busy

busy as hell,
client in the bay

when do we quit
and become farmers?

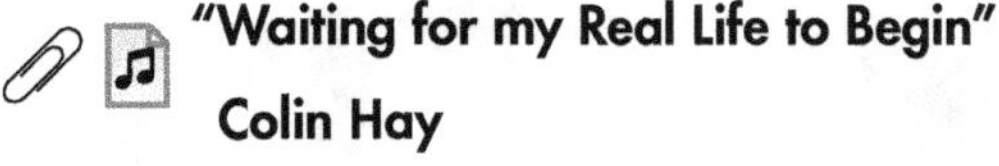

even if i am.

From: chasityrae@gmail.com
To: le_samurai@yahoo.com
Sent: Thursday, April 14, 1:11 p.m.
Subject: Re: busy

soon I hope...

can we have two dogs?
and a pig?
I always wanted a pet pig.

and a huge garden.
with lots of veggies.

mmmmm, and you have to wear
overalls and a cowboy hat.

sounds wonderful.

From: le_samurai@yahoo.com
To: chasityrae@gmail.com
Sent: Thursday, April 14, 1:24 p.m.
Subject: Re: busy

hat and overalls?
hell yeah!

i want to grow everything...

tons of it!
veggies we've never even heard of...

and a barn...
i want a barn too...
and our house has to have a porch...
and a screen door...

i should smoke a pipe too...
when the day is done,
and we're watching the last trace
of blue drain out of the sky...

will you play your guitar for me
in those last moments of the day?
oh, and you have to promise
never to wear shoes...
and have lots of babies...
one for every month...

Love means different things for different people. Anthony described a dizzy, inspired love. Mine meant certainty. For the first time, I felt the difference between knowing love and feeling love, between sincerity and sentiment. I felt it with him. I never told him that then. I was afraid to. Don't laugh, but I saw us in the end of storybooks, the fairytale Emily believed in, the sentiment my coffee-shop friend confessed. Anthony and I were a happily-ever-after. Sure, there where moments Anthony had a tummy ache that would put him in a crabby mood or maybe I would spin out, over-think my actions and question if we were moving too fast—but honestly, it didn't matter then. I was experiencing love instead of trying to figure it all out.

...

From: le_samurai@yahoo.com
To: chasityrae@gmail.com
Sent: Tuesday, April 19, 2:48 p.m.
Subject: the simple life

the simple life you seek
is the one you are living...
to wake up with Gladys,
and flirt with love at work.

we spend so much of our lives
looking to the next moments...
working our asses off to get to that next level...
anticipating what it will be like...

in these moments. in these days.
i am happy. and i am content.
there is heartbreak.
sadness. loneliness.
of course...

but i want to enjoy these times,
need to enjoy these times...
i want to be in love.
beautiful love. crazy fucking love.
the kind of love
that deserves children...
lots and lots of children...
one for every month...
"july! wash your hands before you eat!
april... will you please put a shirt on
before you come to the dinner table..."

Looking back, we were running so fast. Anthony knew we needed to take a step back, and we did—sort of. For weeks we met less, e-mailed three times instead of eight. Drawn in blood, the friendship line gave us time to sort things out in our lives. To get us to where we both wanted to be. Of course we couldn't stop flirting, but we no longer questioned our feelings or desires. We had a secret. No one needed to know how we were feeling. In those moments and in those days, we knew.

chapter ten

our way to fall

"He's such an asshole," I spat at Emily, then turned to Zach. "Did he ever take the time to think about what I wanted? That maybe, just maybe, I'd want to spend my birthday with him?"

Emily and Zach nodded in silence.

"Just because he's telling me in advance," I fumed, "I should be okay with it because he gave me 'time to make other plans.' Eff him. He missed my birthday last year for work, and is going to miss it AGAIN, just so he can visit his grandmother? He couldn't do it ANY other weekend?"

"Your boyfriend is an asshole," Emily stated.

"And he told me over the phone!"

"TOTAL fucker."

"I can't believe he's missing my birthday again. Why would he decide to visit his grandmother that weekend? He didn't even invite me!"

"Complete jerk."

"When's your birthday?" Zach questioned, hoping to settle us so he could continue editing.

"July twentieth!" I yelled.

"Well, it's only June?" he ventured.

"AND," I said, ignoring Zach, "after he gets back from visiting his grandmother, he's going to Hawaii for work!"

Emily and I continued criticizing. Was I hurt? Not really, but kind of. I think I was just more dissatisfied than anything. This was the between-the-lines confirmation I needed, the agreement from friends that Five Year was in fact wrong for me. Sometimes you need that validation from friends. Or, at least I did.

...

From: le_samurai@yahoo.com
To: chasityrae@gmail.com
Sent: Monday, June 13, 11:19 a.m.
Subject: feeling better...

can we have an illicit staircase rendezvous?
something? i need to see you.
like... now...
cause i fucking miss you...

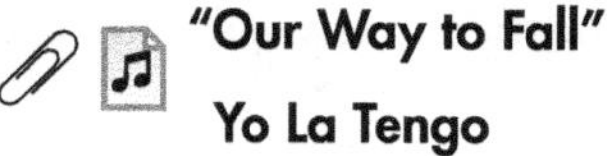

From: chasityrae@gmail.com

To: le_samurai@yahoo.com

Sent: Monday, June 13, 11:20 a.m.

Subject: Re: feeling better...

how about lunch?

We stumbled upon a perfectly grassy hill at the park's entrance and laid out our picnic lunch. The sun warmed my back as we unpacked our sandwiches. It was ideal: a picnic in the middle of a work-filled afternoon.

"Heard you were upset earlier today?"

"Zach told you?"

"Sorry."

"That's okay."

"How you feeling now?"

"Better I guess," I said. Anthony smiled. "Being on a picnic with you helps."

"I thought it might." His smile was saintly. "Do you want to talk about it?"

"I don't know," I fell back into apprehension. "I just feel like I'm wasting my time trying to make my relationship work. I know he and I want different things. I am trying to find my own independence, and strength. I'm tired of this unsatisfied feeling. I want deeper levels of intimacy, conversations, not television over dinner. I don't know. You don't want to hear this."

"I'm still your friend, aren't I?"

"Yeah."

"What do you mean, 'different things?'"

"I want to be married. Married to someone who adores me, can't live without me. Not out of contentment but love. Someone who wants me as his wife—wants *my* children. Someone who wants *me* to come along and visit his grandmother, not just because I want those things, but because he wants them too. Someone who considers me in decisions. I don't know. Maybe I'm asking too much."

"It doesn't sound like too much."

"To him it is. For the past year I've tried to make it work between us, but I feel like love isn't enough sometimes. There needs to be more of a foundation than just love. You know?"

"No. I wish I did."

"I'm sorry. You don't want to hear this. We have enough complications between us. I'm a mess. I guess I just needed to vent."

"Do you feel better?"

"Yes."

"Can we enjoy our picnic now?"

"Yes," still feeling a bit uptight.

I'm glad Anthony changed the subject to work agitations and creative disappointments, blaming his constant tummy ache to stress. I just watched his lips move and his perfect teeth, in love with the words from his mouth to me. His sweet eyes and pervasive smile had me laughing. He could do that—get me to laugh no matter my mood. It was a perfect afternoon. Sitting in the grass, legs crossed, shedding the day's frustrations, my edges softened next to him.

With round full bellies we stretched out in the grass, bathed in sunshine, gazing at the clouds above. He offered an arm for me to rest my head.

"So, now what are you going to do?"

"I don't know. I might take a break from my relationship and be on my own for a while. That was part of the reason I asked you for some space. I need to find my independence. Clear my head. I've been saving a little money… I am in a rut and I think it's time to get out of it." I closed my eyes, took a deep breath. "I need more moments like these."

…

Emily looked concerned. "Chas, there was a call for you at lunch. Your boyfriend has been in a car accident. He's at Cedars Hospital."

chapter eleven

it's okay to think about ending

From: le_samurai@yahoo.com
To: chasityrae@gmail.com
Sent: Wednesday, June 22, 9:45 a.m.
Subject: early hours

sitting down to work,
thinking about you
always thinking about you

in the early hours this morning,
in that place between dreams and consciousness
i held you—
took you in my arms,
felt your hard edge soften
your pace slow to a stop

and it was good.

even if i am.

"It's Okay to Think about Ending"
Earlimart

It's okay, to think about ending.
And it's okay, to not even start
Put it away, wait 'til tomorrow
Put it away, and take care of your heart

I don't know how, but Anthony always found the perfect song to attach.

From: chasityrae@gmail.com
To: le_samurai@yahoo.com
Sent: Wednesday, June 22, 2:07 p.m.
Subject: Re: early morning

thank you.

the past few days have
been overwhelming.
between the two hours of sleep a night,
and changing bandages...
I feel sick.

my boyfriend decided
he didn't want his parents to come
and see him like this...

which means, I am the only help he has.

we've spent the last two days back at the hospital
getting MRIs and CAT scans...
luckily the news has been good.

his stitches won't stop bleeding,
so we have to go to his doctor every twelve hours
for medication to help clot his blood...
right now he's sleeping at the hospital
until his next dose of medication at 5 p.m.

my first break since tues.
I think I'll sneak in a nap
before going back to the hospital.

I wish I had sweet words to send your way.
simple thoughts or phrases to ease your mind.

just know, that I too
am thinking of you.

"Reconstructive surgery just above his eye, a long cut that starts at his eyelid through his eyebrow. It's twenty stitches long."

"Is he okay?" Zach asked as he and I walked for coffee. Zach was a good listener. He had this way of making any hill feel less steep.

"He's pretty banged up—has major cuts on his face from the windshield and burns from the airbags, plus a handful of bruises on his body. I've spent the last week changing bandages, and pulling out small pieces of glass from his forehead. It's absolutely awful. The smell of blood, the crusty ointments..."

"Okay, that's gross."

"Sorry."

"How are you holding up?"

"Like shit. I wish I didn't have to do all of this. I'm not good with blood and needles and stuff."

"Me, neither. I can't imagine."

"Yeah."

"Nothing like a car accident to change your perspective."

"You would think, but after surgery he was more concerned with leaving his computer in the car than finding new perspective. He started listing all the things that were ruined in the accident. His car, iPod, Blackberry, computer..."

"Are you kidding?" Zach turned to look at me seriously.

"No."

"He's lucky he didn't lose one of these." He pointed to his eye, dumbfounded by my response.

"Right."

"Now what are you gonna do?"

"It's not like I can break up with him. Can I?" I was staring at the ground, hoping the pavement would offer up some sort of answer.

"What about Anthony?"

I stopped walking and turned to look at him. "You know?" I had no idea Anthony had confided in Zach. I figured he talked to Jay, but I get it. Zach was someone who knew both of us, a good sounding board.

"Yeah, he needed to tell someone."

"I suppose."

"He really likes you, you know."

"I know." I sighed. "And I really like him."

"So what are you going to do?"

"I have no idea."

"You should talk to Anthony. He's worried about you, and not just for selfish reasons."

Noise interrupted my thoughts as Zach opened the door to the coffee shop.

"I know. I will. Thank you Zach."

"Tall or grande? You're welcome."

...

From: chasityrae@gmail.com
To: le_samurai@yahoo.com
Sent: Thursday, June 30, 6:21 p.m.
Subject: kinda serious...

I started an e-mail early this morning...
it was filled with small talk and frivolous chatter
which only filled the page with nonsense.

even if i am.

so I decided to start over.
to help reassure you,
and tell you again…

I adore you.

it comes in waves
for no reason,
but it fills me.

at night, especially…
when I close my eyes
I imagine you holding me,
wonder how we'd fit together.

and there are moments
when I want to walk into your bay
and kiss you…

and the only thing that gets me
through this, through this time,
is knowing I will have you. someday.
and I don't think about
if we can survive…
I only think about
how nice it will feel
to finally let my guard down

with you.

so, until then...
I will
stay loyal
avoid rumors
and
distance myself...
while slowly gathering strength.

From: le_samurai@yahoo.com
To: chasityrae@gmail.com
Sent: Thursday, June 30, 11:45 p.m.
Subject: Re: kinda serious...

thank you for the e-mail...
i can't begin to explain
how much i needed to hear/read
those words and feelings...
to be reminded, to remember—

it feels like something soft,
something good washing over me...
calming me, restoring me...
bringing me back
to the person i am.

it is a little scary

even if i am.

to feel how much you affect me

...

After the accident, Five Year acted like a spoiled child. Cried when something hurt too much, or sulked when he didn't get his way. He became self-absorbed and focused on material possessions, his career, his appearance. Somehow the accident intensified it all. "Will you still love me if I have a scar on my face?" He lost track of anything he couldn't claim; felt life ripped him off and deserving of more.

I'm not going to lie. Maybe I was looking for faults, but every action disgusted me. I thought he'd wrap his arms around me and confess his love, his devotion to me. I know it's fucked up, but for a brief moment I believed this accident could be our second chance. I tried to right my wrongs by removing bandages wadded and covered with smears of blood and yellow stuff and little pieces of flesh. It was gross. I gagged. Yet, I thought if I took amazing care of him that he'd love me, tell me that he wanted to spend the rest of his life with me—have babies—share everything he had with me...

"Hey, don't forget I am going to Cleveland to visit my grandmother next weekend, then I'm going to Hawaii for work."

"You're still going?" You asshole.

"Of course I'm still going. I've been looking forward to this trip for weeks now."

That was the moment I broke. I couldn't stand him a second longer.

"I'm moving out." I said it before I even thought it.

"What?"

"I can't do this anymore." I pointed back and forth from him to me.

"What do you mean you can't do *this* anymore?" He repeated my gesture.

"I can't be with you. I can't keep pretending that I'm happy."

"What?"

"When I first met you, I wasn't thinking of marriage…"

"There's that word again." He rolled his eyes.

"I didn't think marriage and a family were so important to me, but as I'm slowly finding myself, these things are important—you say you understand but you don't. It's not just a phase I am going through. I want more."

"Why are you doing this to me? Especially now."

"Doing this to *you*? I didn't realize what a selfish jackass you can be. This car accident has only made you worse. I'm tired of changing bandages. And, I am tired of compromising. At the end of the road, you and I want different things. I see that now. We are not what I want anymore."

Like an angered three-year-old, he started crying before I could say another word. "I knew this would happen. I knew you'd do this to me."

He kept babbling, completely irrational. Every redeeming word, thought, or sentence I uttered was followed with a shout of disapproval. There was nothing left to chew. He was done listening. I was fighting a war I knew I would lose. I left the room as he lay crying on our bed, still yelling.

...

I slept on the couch. Five Year took the bedroom. I didn't remind him of my decision to move out, or that I was actively looking. Why bother. It was hard enough to keep the peace throughout our home. If we did converse, it was brief. The word love was no longer used. I worked extra hours avoiding him. He worked extra hours avoiding me.

On lunch breaks I would tour new apartments and areas throughout the city, imagining my new home. I'd forgotten what it was like to live my own life. Maybe I never knew, but the thrill of looking for a place had me hopeful—heartbroken, but hopeful. Five years together no longer mattered. It was time for fresh starts and clean slates.

chapter twelve

shelter

Anthony kept his word. We kept it at bay. No secret rendezvous, only brief e-mails and a couple of phone calls. I had been so busy playing nurse, and then finding an apartment, that I was preoccupied. Two weeks was all it took. Two weeks and I missed Anthony.

I called, pleading, "Meet me in the stairwell?"

...

"Two blocks from work!" Nudging him, I added, "Come on, indulge my enthusiasm."

"A new home, eh? That's exciting." He didn't really indulge.

"Yeah, we'll see. Fingers crossed."

"Did you come up with any birthday plans yet?"

"Not really. I still have a couple of days to think about it. I might have dinner with friends. How about you? How are you? Since the accident it feels like we haven't spent much time together."

"We haven't," he said halfhearted. His hand drifted to his tummy.

"Sorry," I said, lowering my tone to match his.

"That's okay. I'm okay. Work's been crazy lately." He sounded upset.

"Is something wrong?"

"No, not really. Just some health stuff. I haven't been feeling very good. I didn't want to tell you. You already have a lot going on..."

"Really? Is it your stomach again?"

"Yeah, the stomach aches are getting worse," he mumbled. "Umm, this is kind of awkward but I'm bleeding when I take a number two." We both sat there, mute for a moment. "I went to my doctor last week, and he scheduled a colonoscopy."

"Oh." I am a jerk, sometimes. I am. I should have reached out sooner.

"I get this feeling it's something serious. Too many stomachaches in a row."

I noticed how his hand settled on his stomach for comfort.

"Maybe it's an ulcer or hemorrhoids or something?"

"Maybe."

"Are you scared?" I looked him directly in the eyes, trying to see if I should be, too.

"I don't know. Kind of." He now examined his hand to his tummy.

"When's the colonoscopy?"

"On Monday."

"Do you have a ride? I can take you. My boyfriend leaves on Saturday to visit his grandma. I could probably get out of work?" I explained this all in one long breath.

"No, that's okay. I think Jay can pick me up."

I felt a little disappointed.

"If you need anything, will you please call me?"

"Yes."

"Promise?"

"Yes. I promise."

"Can I have a hug?"

"Always." He grabbed me tightly.

...

From: chasityrae@gmail.com

To: le_samurai@yahoo.com

Sent: Monday, July 18, 6:04 p.m.

Subject: you're not here, but I'm sending an e-mail

my LEAST favorite thing?
is when you are not here,
and at the doctor's...

I am sending you all the love

and strength my body can offer...
can you feel it?
damn I miss you...

I wish I could hold your hand right now,
and tell you
everything
is going to be okay.

...

Anthony called, still groggy. In one long run-on sentence he explained the colonoscopy. From the anesthesia countdown to the monitor presenting his colon, he was awake during the entire process as the camera looked for obstructions. He said they found a lump and took a biopsy.

"You okay?" I questioned.

"I am now that I've heard your voice." His voice was sleepy and sweet. "Jay's here, so can I call you later tonight?"

"Yeah..."

"Okay."

"Anthony?"

"Yeah?"

"I miss you."

"I miss you more."

...

It was reassuring to hear his soft voice on the other end of the line. I told him I got the house. "The one two blocks from work. I move in August." I described the yard for Gladys, the perfectly square layout, and the pink exterior. He told me I looked sexy in pink. We talked until one in the morning, eager, playful, and hopeful for days ahead. I said so. He said so. Half-awake, half-asleep, we joked about running away for my birthday.

"Weren't we supposed to elope in Mexico?" we said in unison.

...

From: le_samurai@yahoo.com
To: chasityrae@gmail.com
Sent: Tuesday, July 19, 9:07 a.m.
Subject: shelter

it still amazes me
how far down some roads
we have traveled,
while there are so many other roads
we have not even touched...

staying up on the phone,
talking to obscene hours,

even if i am.

and nearly falling asleep
ear to ear with each other...
it is something we should have done
a long, long time ago...

it seems as though
to make up for what
we cannot do together,
we take the things we can do,
and run with them as far
as they can be taken...

exploding within our limitations...
the song i am sending
is one that brought us to mind,
one that made me think
that perhaps it is a good thing
we are both taking on great difficulties
at the same time in our lives...
similarity?

"you will shelter me, my love
and i... i will shelter you...
i will shelter you..."

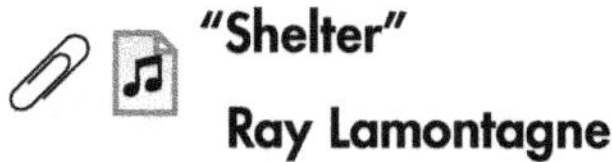

From: chasityrae@gmail.com
To: le_samurai@yahoo.com
Sent: Tuesday, July 19, 12:21 p.m.
Subject: similarities

the "great difficulties"
we are both enduring

may get uncomfortable at times...
may make the "us" we've created,
and so desperately hung on to, difficult.

but I do believe it is the similarities that will
bring us closer...
to the end of the roads
we have yet to experience.

and through it all I will secretly wish
for another late night conversation...

because those moments with you,
are simply beautiful.

even if i am.

From: le_samurai@yahoo.com
To: chasityrae@gmail.com
Sent: Tuesday, July 19, 2:34 p.m.
Subject: the heels of happiness

the challenges...
the similarities...

yes, i think those are the things
that bring us together unconsciously,
that will bring us together ultimately...

it freaks me out a bit
to talk in that tense...
the future...
i know it freaks you out too...

and besides,
it is so much better to live it
as it unfolds than it is
to talk about what we expect it to be...

and i can feel your fear,
that we are growing too fast...
that if you loosen the leash
just a little bit,
we will run completely
out of control...

shelter

and i know you feel,
that with every inch
you and i sink deeper into each other,
the delirious pleasure
of surrender…
of hope…
of love…

but on the heels of happiness
comes the fear of having let in too much
confusion…
complication…
second guesses…

know that i am here.
for you.
when you are ready.
if you are ready.

no assumptions.
no expectations.

with hope.
and fears.
but mostly hope…

and love.

even if i am.

lots of fucking love...

...

Running downstairs to his bay, I couldn't move fast enough.

"What did the doctor say?"

He hesitated, filling his lungs with air, then puffed out one big breath.

"They found a malignant tumor on my colon."

chapter thirteen

happy birthday

ANTHONY, CAN WE GO BACK TO THAT MOMENT? CAN YOU tell me again what you said after, "They found a malignant tumor on my colon," because I have no idea.

I assume the details of your conversation with the doctor. My mind just repeated the word tumor. Tumor. Tumor. I didn't know what to say so I told you my mother has cancer. I have no idea why I said it. I thought it would be helpful. How was I supposed to react when you told me they found a tumortumortumor?

I think people give hugs. I'm sorry, I gave you a pep talk instead. Trying to sound hopeful instead of random. I said, "You'll beat this. I know you will. I promise you will. You're only thirty." I felt like a cheerleader.

I ended up hugging you. Not just any hug, mind you, but a hug that I believed could cure. Asthma. Arthritis. Even cancer. I think you did too, because you squeezed as hard as you could.

"Fuck." You tried not to cry. "I have cancer."

"We'll beat this. I promise."

...

You left work early. I muddled through the rest of the day in a fog, and then went home promptly at 6:00 p.m. The house was empty except for Gladys, sleeping on the couch. I must have watched her sleep for hours before I wrapped my arms around her tired body and cried. I cried through the evening, sobbing through my TV dinner, slipped on PJs, and then cried myself to sleep.

I cried at the thought of losing you, babe. I cried at the thought of never having you. I wished I was smarter, knew the right words to say—that I didn't say the word cancer. I wished I was stronger emotionally and would've left Five Year sooner. I wished life wasn't so fucked up and complicated, wasn't so much bullshit. I wished we didn't have to pretend we were anything but what we were. In love.

I wished I would've gone to your bay and kissed you all the times I wanted to, made out with you in the stairwell. I wished many things.

I woke to the sound of my cell phone. Thought it a dream to hear your voice on the other end telling me to come outside.

"What?"

"Just go outside already."

"But I'm sleeping. I'm in my PJs."

"There's a surprise for you outside your door."

I stumbled out of bed, slid on slippers. "This better be good. What time is it anyway?" I swung open my front door.

At exactly midnight with two pints of ice cream and a single candle illuminating the inside of your truck, I saw you.

"Come on, get in," you yelled out the window. "It's not right to celebrate your birthday alone."

I climbed in.

"Okay, which flavor, Cherry Garcia or Chunky Monkey?"

I followed all the rules, man's, God's, my parents'—I no longer cared about consequences as I crawled over to the driver's side. Like a child in your lap, I kissed you. Hard. Unlike I'd ever kissed anyone. Ever.

"Don't let go of me, even if I ask you to," I muttered in between skin and lips. Devouring you with kisses, ice cream melting in the passenger's seat.

"Happy birthday." You started to sing as you grabbed me, not letting go.

chapter fourteen

no woman no cry

My cafe friend asked me if I felt as certain about Anthony as she did with her new love, if I felt as giddy and girly. It's a question I hesitated to answer. I've been asked it before and God only knows why I can't answer it honestly. I simply say yes. I give a one-word response. It was a superficial answer and I wish I could revise myself. It's not that the question is intrusive; it's just too personal. I have needed five years to understand the depth of what that question means.

It's why the rest of the story is easier to tell when I imagine you, babe, at my side finishing my sentences like old times. Because to tell the passionate, difficult truth, I need you to help me; reminding me that our love is a universal human experience and it deserves to be opened up and shared.

So here we go, Anthony. I'm counting on you to listen, and to help me finish what we started together, five years ago.

even if i am.

...

From: le_samurai@yahoo.com
To: chasityrae@gmail.com
Sent: Friday, July 22, 5:36 p.m.
Subject: full

you...
sigh
(cue heart swoon)

an interesting week we've had,
with ups and downs...
late nights
closeness...

that's what it is...
a closeness
much closer than before...

don't know when we broke through
whatever it was we had to get through,
but you feel...
amazing
unguarded...

or rather,
i feel

like
i am in your heart...
deep in your heart

Of the conversations, it's the little ones you look back on. The ones you wish you could go back to and have again. Maybe the conversations don't even have real importance or hold much weight, but you remember it. It marks a time. A place. A feeling. You remember the words and the sentiments. I remember the voice I used to comfort you, Anthony, and I certainly remember my fears. However, in this one conversation, it's the words, "what if," that I remember most.

...

"Come closer," I cooed. I was sitting on the top step of our stairs with my arms opened to embrace him. "What'd they say?" Trying to get Anthony's attention, I shook his body while I embraced him. "You okay?"

"Yeah, I'm fine. Telling my roommates was difficult, harder than I imagined. They were sweet, strong, supportive but then they started talking about how we're like a family in this house, and how everyone will be here for me—take care of me... It made me sad and scared."

"Why scared?"

"Scared I'm going to let them down somehow. Seems foolish, but... what if I won't be able to take care of them?"

There it was. Maybe we were thinking about other what ifs, but this was the first.

"What do you mean?"

"What if I am too sick to be their friend—what if I'm too sick when they need me?"

Anthony fiddled with his fingernails, and his hands shook and I knew he was scared to talk such nonsense but I thought he was absurd and so selfless.

"I think you're absurd."

Neither of us knew what to say. Instead silence filled the space between an exhaled sigh as he hid his face in my neck, rubbed his nose into my hair. He did that when he needed comfort, and I would press my cheek against his forehead, nuzzling back for the same sense of relief.

"My boyfriend gets home tonight…" We both sat upright. "I'm afraid to move out. I have no idea why, but I feel trapped, too weak to leave, or stir up conflict." I kept barfing out words like *unhappy*, *unsatisfied*, and *uncomfortable*. Any word I could conjure starting in *un*. "Most of all I feel uneasy. I'm not a cheater. I don't feel like I've cheated."

"You haven't," he said, snickering. "Trust me. I know."

"No, seriously." I elbowed him, half-grinning. "I need to tell him this is really happening. I'm moving out. I owe him that. I need to tell him he's not a horrible person, just not the person for me. How do I say that? After five years how do you tell the person you love that it's simply not enough. I'm scared of his reaction. He acts like a child these days. I don't know why this is so hard. I'm scared I guess."

"You've said, 'I'm scared,' a couple times now."

"I know. I know. Sorry. This probably seems so trivial."

"You are far from trivial. I am here, whenever, or however you need me to be, even if only a friend. I thought we've worked that out by now."

"I know." I nestled into his shoulder with a soft, slow exhale. "Then there's you, sweet, snuggly you." I loved the way he tickled the tip of his nose against my neck. "Are you going to tell your mom tonight?"

"I'll try."

"Anthony, you've told friends. You've told your brothers. It's time."

"I know." He didn't want to talk about it anymore. I don't blame him. "Okay, we'd better get back to work. Meet me in my truck later?"

"Yes."

He headed to the sixth floor while I stood on the seventh.

"Are you still scared?" I yelled down the stairwell.

"Trying not to be. You?"

"Terrified."

even if i am.

...

From: le_samurai@yahoo.com

To: chasityrae@gmail.com

Sent: Wednesday, July 27, 10:22 a.m.

Subject: i couldn't attach the song i wanted to send with this...

and that sucks because it was perfect

i am scared
of being scared...
and so,
i am not.

even if i am.

for too much of my life,
at the worst times, some random times
and inevitably embarrassing times,
my hands have shaken...

despite me.
my efforts to focus.
calm.
steady...

FUCK!

no woman no cry

and it is a sad betrayal
when your body gives up your mind,
shows that which you would conceal,
that which you cannot…

but something good
has come out of it…

and that is,
i know i still must act.
must push through it,
must do whatever it is.

fear is familiar.
and so,
when it comes
i know what to do.

"my fear is my only courage
so i have to push on through…"
—bob marley

i know…
i can't believe i just quoted bob marley either,
but it came to mind,
and even if i sound like
a college freshman…
it helps the point.

even if i am.

despite your efforts
to illustrate the contrary,
i don't think you are fearful.

i think you are bold.
and i think you are beautiful.
i think you are bold and beautiful.
(oh christ, i'm losing it...)

but there is something inside of you,
something i have seen:
a strength. steadiness. courage.

as opaque as you are.
it is easy to see.

perhaps you are scared now,
frozen by the fear you feel
because you don't know
how to handle it...

fear is not familiar for you.

we are defined by
who we are in crisis...
you are overwhelmed.
so quit your fucking whining

and do something about it.

something amazing.
because that is who you are.
that is what i see.

...

Five Year returned from his trip visiting his grandmother in Cleveland. He showered me with guilt gifts, inquired about my birthday and the details of my week. I gave stock replies, and then my automated response turned attention to his travels. He described Cleveland, his childhood home, his grandmother's appearance. I never met his grandmother, but she sounded sweet. I knew very little of his home and childhood in Cleveland. His stories were new and interesting. It was good to see him, a forgotten comfort in our lazy love. We kissed, hugged, conversed like old friends, finished each other's sentences, and then laughed. I felt content.

I sat on the edge of the bed and searched for the courage while he removed dirty clothes from his suitcase. I knew this would be our last goodbye. I thought of your e-mail, your expressions, moreover, your strength.

I am scared of being scared... and so, I am not. Even if I am.

even if i am.

...

You never did tell me how the phone call went, but I imagined you pacing the room, rehearsing the conversation a dozen times while contemplating your mother's response. Knowing you, you thought about everything to say, extremely careful in selecting words. I wouldn't be surprised if you even wrote it down. Yes, you definitely wrote it down in that green notebook you always carried, highlighting key points, outlining needed details. Taking your time with the placement of each word. Likely your mind raced, listing things you should have done, should have finished or started. I bet you even blamed yourself for getting cancer. Somehow it was your fault. Persuaded yourself you needed to apologize to her first. You practiced your replies, your assurance.

Weeks' worth of conversations had gone by and now it was time to tell her. You told me that you only cried once when you thought of telling her. You had a malignant tumor, and you hadn't shed a tear. Maybe no one told you there is strength in crying. Though, I know that this moment, the simple thought of telling your mother made you sob. Uncontrollably. You wept. You wept for her fears, for her concerns, lamented your own pressures, awkward emotions, uncomfortable skin. Phone in hand. You were scared. Your hands shook while you dialed the number. This I am sure of.

I am scared of being scared...and so, I am not. Even if I am.

"Hi, Mama."

"Anthony," she sung, "it's good to hear your voice. How are you?"

Swallowing your tears, "I'm okay."

"Just okay?"

"I have something I need to tell you…"

chapter fifteen

jealousy rides with me

Before I met Anthony, everything I knew of love was a long way off. I thought love was complex and compound; like one of those word problems in math, usually involving a train's speed, that no one could solve.

"Stage 3 colon cancer."

"Out of?"

"Four."

"Shit."

You know, thinking back, that was the moment. After Anthony was diagnosed, our relationship changed. Love became singular. One times one equaled one. Basic math, no word problems or freight trains. We were beyond intimate. It would only seem like a reasonable progression, love. But there was something about it—a singular strength of feeling. Something I hadn't experienced in previous relationships. Sounds crazy, cliché even. I can get outside of myself sometimes, but I truly felt Anthony was my missing piece. My Shel Silverstein's "Big O." The piece that makes you whole. The circle that teaches the triangle to soften its edges and roll alongside. The "O" that brings out the best in you, surrounds you with love, the piece that completes you and tells you, "You'll be all right, because I'm by your side."

My Big O. My train home.

...

"Hey, I need your opinion," Anthony said causally as we walked to get lunch.

"Okay."

"Since you're going to be the mother of my children..." He poked my side. I giggled and squirmed. "I think we should store sperm before starting chemo."

I tickled back. "I think that's an excellent idea. What do we have to do?"

I know. This is an absurd question to be asking someone you've not had sex with. Then again, love is absurd.

"There is a clinic that stores your sperm until you need it. Weird, right? Like rented storage space. I guess I just have to go down to the clinic and, ummm, put a specimen—or 'friends' as I like to call them—in a storage container." He wiggled his finger mimicking a friend swimming, and tickled me again.

"Sounds kinky," I taunted. "I say store as much as you can. Then we have the comfort of knowing there's always the chance for a family. If I know anything about you, that's pretty important." Like a mischievous child, I quickly ran ahead. "Plus, if we plan to have a boy for each month..."

"Boys, huh?" He rushed to catch me, grabbed my waist and threw me over his shoulder as we stumbled down the street laughing. "First, we should probably have sex."

"To see if it even fits." I giggled upside down.

"Hell, I'd be happy to touch your boobs."

...

From: chasityrae@gmail.com
To: le_samurai@yahoo.com
Sent: Thursday, July 28, 4:11 p.m.
Subject: mother of your children...

do you think it's strange...
that you said that with such
confidence and certainty?
and I simply agreed.

From: le_samurai@yahoo.com
To: chasityrae@gmail.com
Sent: Thursday, July 28, 5:18 p.m.
Subject: Re: mother of your children...

yeah...
we're weird...

even if i am.

doesn't one usually come
WAY WAY WAY before the other???

we're definitely
on a weird wavelength...

From: chasityrae@gmail.com
To: le_samurai@yahoo.com
Sent: Thursday, July 28, 6:36 p.m.
Subject: Re: mother of your children...

strangest relationship in history...
and yet there is something
words can't explain.

...

One day not long after the diagnosis, I managed to keep my mind occupied with work projects and packing. My office phone rang and I hurried to answer, expecting Anthony's sweet voice calling to tell me the story of putting "friends" in storage.

"Hey, Chas."

"Oh, hey, Zach."

"Do you know where Anthony is?"

"He left for the uh, the doctor earlier today. What's up?"

"Oh, I wanted to catch up with him before I left work."

"Sorry, but you just missed him. You could try his cell?"

"No worries."

Hearing disappointment in Zach's voice I offered, "Hey, I was thinking about going for a walk after work? Care to join me?"

"Would love to."

If I had to guess, Zach had a crush on me. I am female and blonde and have boobs; the basic elements of Zach's type. I inherited my mother's looks and tendency to flirt. I'm the Midwest girl Zach grew up adoring in Chicago. We liked to chat about movies—he liked blockbusters, I preferred art house. We gossiped about work scandals and trash-talked our latest projects. But honestly, apart from any common ground or crush he might have had on me, I think Zach liked me because he had a man-crush on Anthony. He wanted to fit into the cool crowd and Anthony was, well, cool. He'd find reasons for the three of us to go for coffee walks and lunch breaks. We didn't know it then, but Zach would become our third wheel. He'd become our crutch and the first person to ever take our picture together.

"Have you ever hiked to the top of the canyon and seen the view of Hollywood?" I asked.

"Nope."

"Really?" He shook his head in confirmation. "Well, then, it's your lucky day. We are hiking to the top." I raised my fist and marched onward. "When you called looking for Anthony, you sounded a little bummed. How are you holding up?"

"Like shit, but getting through it. I'm still trying to grasp the fact that one of my best friends has cancer, and there is absolutely nothing I can do about it. I feel helpless, and I don't want to cheapen my time with him talking about work."

"Talking about work is helping more than you know. Trust me."

I don't need to go on about the importance of friends, but it's hard not to here. Their distractions, even work, made Anthony hugely happy.

...

I guess I just had one of those wishful-thinking moments, babe, that everything was great between us. I flashed my bright glowing smile, my immediate reaction whenever you caught me off guard—you had that way. Yet, you said nothing as you exited the elevator. Just walked by, gave me the cold shoulder. You never acted like this before, so I knew something was wrong. I dialed your office number and let the phone ring until you answered.

"No friendly morning banter?"

"Not in the mood."

"Why?"

"I ran into to Zach and heard about your hike. I don't know... Sort of irritating."

"What?"

"You can go to the movies, hang out, and hike with Zach, but we remain behind closed doors. This—whatever *this* is, it's not working. It feels like I'm repeating an all-too-familiar cycle of sneaking around."

"I have no idea where this is coming from."

"Of course you don't."

You hung up the phone. You're a jerk sometimes.

...

From: le_samurai@yahoo.com
To: chasityrae@gmail.com
Sent: Monday, August 1, 1:57 p.m.
Subject: yuck!

i wish i could unzip this feeling,
take it off like a jacket,
and fucking burn it.

fuck.

i want to be able
to let go of it...

have fun with zach.
walk up the fucking canyon,
and look at the fucking view...

even if i am.

too much
on my
fucking
mind.

felt one way this morning…
turned quickly into something else.

fucking sucks.

me.
i have
to fucking focus.
on me.

strength.
center.
breathe.

and…

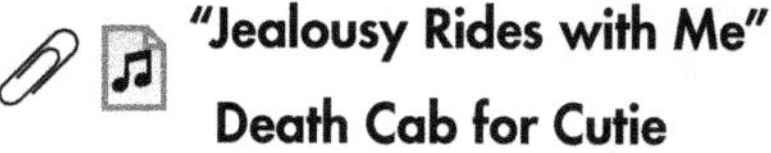

…

It's a part of our story I wish to forget, a splinter in my perfect memory of us. We weren't perfect—no couple is. I get that. But, this fight seemed frivolous. And I hated arguing in our stairwell at work.

"YES. You. Have. To. Focus. On. You. No question. I need to do the same." Do you remember? You came back with a long-winded dialogue about ending our "shadowed" relationship. You explained your jealousy towards Zach, expressing "unhealthy feelings that hindered your mental and physical health." We never even sat down on a step. You stood to disagree. I stood to reassure.

"Am I supposed to walk away and not want to see you?" I urged, talking slowly to emphasize each word. "Because as much as you need to focus on your health, I won't let you go. I. Am. Not. Walking. Away." You kept blathering on about ending, as I kept pleading, "It breaks me that you feel like this. I want to tell you things, hug you, yell at you, whatever it takes to make these feelings go away."

Maybe you were right. Maybe we were chasing our tails. Maybe it was best for us to just lay off a little while. Then we could work it out some other time, when we were happy and healthy, without situations and complications. You could go off and heal. I could go and…

The lack of what to do nearly sent me to my knees. "What happens when secrets and 'shadowed' relationships *are* worth fighting for? Then what? Then what do you do?"

"We can't do this anymore. I have cancer." You looked hopelessly at me.

The words burnt my skin. Baby, I knew what you where thinking. I was thinking it too; and maybe we should've talked about it then, but we can't change that. We can't go back. I don't know what it is about the word *cancer* that sends everyone's mind branching to an assortment of what-ifs. But let's be honest, there is only one what-if that stands ahead of the line, and everyone was afraid to say it around you. And I wasn't going to let you walk away because you were afraid of it, too.

So, what if you did die? I would be alone. That didn't mean you needed to leave me now.

chapter sixteen

jóga

Babe, I couldn't stand it. Everything changed so fast. Four days had passed, and we were completely disconnected. I didn't care if I was right or wrong or if I flirted with Zach or if you were being an asshole, or if you were scared of the what-if. I just wanted you closer.

I typed the e-mail a dozen times. It started with an apology. I reread it; the words trite and trivial. I was trying to find the perfect lines. Hours passed as I listened to a dozen songs scrutinizing each lyric. Nothing was perfect. I needed something perfect. But that's it: love isn't perfect. You know that. It breaks your heart. The storybooks are bullshit. There is no knight in shining…

And just like that, I knew exactly what to send.

even if i am.

From: chasityrae@gmail.com
To: le_samurai@yahoo.com
Sent: Friday, August 5, 4:59 p.m.
Subject: the movie is moonstruck

loretta I love you...
and not like they told you love is

and I didn't know this either,
but love don't make things nice...
it ruins everything
it breaks your heart
it makes things a mess...

WE aren't here to make things perfect
the snowflakes are perfect
the stars are perfect...
not us
NOT US!

WE are here to ruin ourselves
and to break our hearts
and to love the wrong people
and DIE!

I mean the storybooks are bullshit!
now will you come upstairs with me
and GET INTO MY BED!

...

Like an early '90s movie staring Cher and Nicholas Cage, the ones whose every line you've memorized—I didn't even tell Anthony I was coming. Yet there he stood in our stairwell waiting to say, "I fucking love you."

"But that's my line." I smiled through the words.

We kissed and fondled for the first time since my birthday. He detailed his morning visit to the radiologist, and his treatment strategy; for the next four weeks radiation every morning, while consuming chemo pills three times a day. I confirmed I had started packing. Our entire conversation fit between a breath and another kiss.

...

From: le_samurai@yahoo.com
To: chasityrae@gmail.com
Sent: Friday, August 5, 6:44 p.m.
Subject: Re: moonstruck

this quote was perfect...
just my kind of thing
does that mean you are coming over tonight?

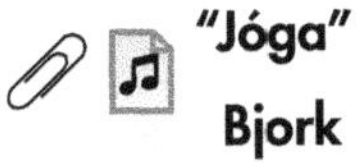

"Jóga"
Bjork

chapter seventeen

i want you

THERE WAS A TIME I CONSIDERED MYSELF TO BE A SMART aleck, a personality trait I wasn't necessarily proud of. People called me a pessimist. But here's the thing: I wasn't pessimistic about cancer. I'd already seen its face—in my mother's cervical cancer and my grandfather's prostate cancer. Hell, Gladys my dog has cancer. Cancer is a half-full glass.

Anthony's treatment was planned to be straightforward, logical, and optimistic. It consisted of a regimen of chemo pills and radiation for six weeks, followed by colorectal surgery in November, which would remove any existing tumors. After surgery, he would face one more round of follow-up chemo, then remission. Cancer sounded simple. A, B, C, and then happily-ever-after.

He packed for a summer trip to Maine as I crammed boxes for my new life in a pink house. Time was on our side. I knew nothing about colon cancer, but I didn't need to. Ahead of us were summer, pills, radiation, dates, movies, friends, fun, love. It was the summer of possibilities as we held onto hope.

...

From: le_samurai@yahoo.com
To: chasityrae@gmail.com
Sent: Tuesday, August 9, 2:04 p.m.
Subject: maine

we just got DSL at the house in maine,
so i will be able to write
(and hopefully read)
e-mails on a regular basis.
writing to you is very much
like writing a journal:
open, descriptive, consistent.

i am planning on bringing
both my digital still camera
and my video camera
to document the trip.
looking forward to showing you
just how retarded my family is,
how beautiful the lake is,
and just where and when
i would have wished you could be.

going to read lance armstrong
i think his book is just the thing
i need to read before jumping
into radiation and chemotherapy.

6 p.m. sharp.
let's get the helloutahere!

...

"You can hug me if you want to." I grabbed Anthony's waist before he finished the word hug.

"Okay, I better head to the airport." His arms left mine.

"Miss me."

I know, I said it wrong.

...

From: le_samurai@yahoo.com
To: chasityrae@gmail.com
Date: Tuesday, August 10, 1:12 p.m.
Subject: in the tradition

of being seventh graders,
i want you to know
that i miss you already...

and i send you

even if i am.

all the strength i have
to help you with your heart,
and your move...

...

I owned very little, only a small U-Haul's worth, but I packed boxes labeled kitchen, bedroom, and bath, taping cardboard and wrapping glasses as if I were moving across the country. Some dishes, a coffee table, bookshelf, books, clothes, and Gladys were the requirements. I packed only known belongings, and left any co-purchases Five Year might question, including Kala, our cat. She scratched him whenever he tried to hold her. I smiled at her curled on the couch, knowing she would be the first to comfort him home.

Okay, maybe I left her out of spite.

Friends dollied furniture to the moving truck. As the packing progressed, I felt fragments of regret while examining framed photos. *What have I done? How did I let it get this far?* I thought about the first time I met Five Year, the years, the moments. The day I moved into this apartment, his apartment. Our anniversaries, holidays...

"Come on, you're slowing down." Zach nudged my shoulder as I sighed. He crouched on the floor next to me and examined a celebrated snapshot of a past Christmas.

"I can't believe I am really doing this," I said, shaking my head.

"Me, neither."

"Really?" I said, stunned.

"Really. It feels like you've been talking about this move forever. And, well, I thought you'd stay with him, even though you were unhappy. You kept giving it a chance, and it seemed like an easier option than starting over."

That's me, my usual pattern of always trying to work it out.

Zach grabbed the photo and placed it into the box. "You can't change your mind now. All the boxes are in the U-Haul and I'm not about to unpack them for doubts."

"He's going to want to blame someone for my leaving."

"Like himself?"

"I honestly think he did the best he could."

"And yet he was still so selfish."

"And now so am I." I double taped the last box and labeled SELFISH STORAGE. "Time to be selfish."

"How does it feel?" Zach asked.

"Hopeful."

"Okay, truck is ready." He grabbed the last box.

I kissed Kala on the head and whispered, "Be good to him."

chapter eighteen

songs i listened to five years ago

I GO TO A SUPPORT GROUP NOW, FIVE YEARS LATER. I NEVER really wanted to go, but I thought it would help and people kept telling me I needed to talk to someone instead of looking at old photographs and listening to remembered songs. There are a handful of people in the group, all of us sharing our stories of love and loss. They tell me it's good to write down how I am feeling to help me deal with it all, and trust me, there is a lot to deal with. I've been writing, but every time I do, I don't know what to write. I told the group that. Afterward a woman came up to me, placed her hand on my shoulder and said, stop writing *about* him and start writing *to* him.

chapter nineteen

i melt with you

I WAS FLUSTERED. I PACED AIMLESSLY IN MY OFFICE AND dialed your extension four times before you finally picked up, babe. "What the hell took you so long?" It was Monday, our first day back at work together in over a week. I came in early because I hadn't seen you in a lifetime. "Meet me in the stairwell."

We didn't talk, just kissed. Uncontrollably.

...

From: le_samurai@yahoo.com
To: chasityrae@gmail.com
Sent: Thursday, August 18, 3:17 p.m.
Subject: smile

when you smile at me,
holding it just a little longer

even if i am.

than you normally would...
it just about makes me melt.

i know i'm not being chatty,
and i'm sorry...
but it's mostly because
i'm trying to jump back
into the workflow around here...
(feeling a little like a waste)

and i'm also trying to figure out
how my body is dealing with
all this new stuff
i'm putting into it...

freakedout.

tonight is for you,
fun in any form you want it—
i'd love to see your house?

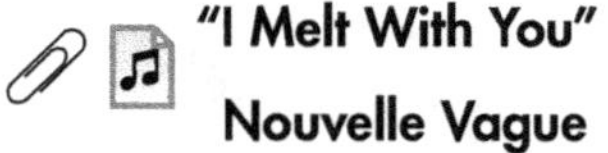

...

It's probably my favorite memory; the one of us touring my 500-square-foot home for the first time. Seems so long ago, doesn't it, babe? The memory is difficult to label and file. It's bold. It's the memory that keeps wanting to be remembered. You do that—you have a way of making our memories unforgettable.

"This is my bathroom." I had only an AM radio, a full size bed, and a few half-full boxes thrown about. As we moved through the mini maze, we ignored the belongings that were tolerantly waiting to be shown their new place. "This is my kitchen." Standing in the middle of the room, we circled ourselves. That's all the room allowed. I showed you the pantry I loved. Do you remember how big it was? "When on earth would I need that much space for food? Isn't it incredible?"

"You really are starting over, aren't you?"

Gazing at the clutter of possessions, I said, "I am." A long exhale escaped me. "Tell me something good?"

Your eyes met mine and you said, "You're simply beautiful." I know I blushed as you grabbed my hand, led me to the only furniture in the house, a bed full of towels and laundry. You pushed the disorder aside, laid me softly on the mattress and removed your shirt. You didn't hesitate. Caught between the felt and the imagined, desire broke any apprehension. I unbuttoned mine. Your hands moved like waves over me. You untied the knots of my legs with your kisses and lips. Not a word spoken between us. There was little to say. Everything had led up to this point. I knew how you felt, and there was nothing more to reveal. I wrapped my arms around your neck, swaying my hips. I wanted to bury myself in you, get lost with you. My embrace alternately soft, then fierce. Laundry crumpled between us. I held my breath until you finished. *I'll stop the world and melt with you.*

...

You attached a picture of Odilon Redon's *The Barque* with the e-card you sent. Two people on a boat in the darkness caught between a description and a dream. You wrote:

i wanted to find a different way
to say good morning,
because this feels like a different day...

waking up with you
after a beautiful evening together,
was absolutely lovely...

a.

Beyond the visible, beyond the evident, that night I staggered into the direction I was afraid of. All the roads I had traveled, relationships I had twisted my heart for—they felt like part of another lifetime, when love was melancholy and the road was full of mud. I was burned out from exhaustion. And then I turned around and there you stood, just beyond the visible. I didn't have time to get my mind straight. I was, very late that night and in the morning hours, caught by you beside me, on me, in me, behind me.

"When you wake up, is it me you want to see?"

"Forever."

I tried my best to get out of bed, but your kiss convinced me otherwise.

chapter twenty

ache for you

It was the dawn of sleepovers, endless hours spent tangled in sheets, exploring our bodies, sampling positions. From the first night of intimacy and every night thereafter, we cuddled, groped, spooned, and adored. We couldn't get enough of each other. (Okay, at least I couldn't get enough.) I was your blanket, and you were mine. I wanted to confess, confide my love in the middle of orgasm. With sex I loved wholly. With sex I gave everything.

However—a HUGE, catastrophic, a something-everyone-should-know-before-getting-involved-in-a-serious-relationship "however"—there was also the lack of sleep. I never thought about sleep. The physical act of sleep, the simple REM stage needed daily. I worried about parents and friends; I wondered about compatibility and foundation, sex and intimacy. But sleep? Anthony, you were the WORST sleeper of all time.

even if i am.

There. I said it. Sleeping with you, disastrous. Disastrous might even be a bit of an understatement. Sleeping side by side with you was just plain terrible. You tossed and turned, adjusting and repositioning. Kicked off blankets. Rolled yourself into a human burrito with the blankets. God forbid if the blankets were tucked into any crease around the mattress. Your body was fiery hot, and your toes cold and clammy. Your feet hung over the edge of my bed, persuading you to angle from corner to farthest corner leaving me only the upper edge, coverless. Hallelujah if I still had a pillow by sunrise. Sex was simple, wonderful. Sleep, dreadful.

...

From: le_samurai@yahoo.com
To: chasityrae@gmail.com
Sent: Friday, August 26, 9:41 a.m.
Subject: me first...

feeling awake,
productive, and good...

expecting to fall asleep
where i'm standing
sometime around 11 a.m....

last night was beautiful...
and then uncomfortable,

disorienting, and ultimately hilarious...

so...
next time we have a sleepover,
can we go to my house?
where it's quiet,
the bed doesn't cut off my ankles,
and we're not being serenaded to sleep
by the traffic on highland blvd.?

p.s. it was still wonderful. sort of.

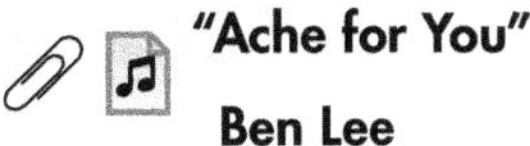
"Ache for You"
Ben Lee

From: chasityrae@gmail.com
To: le_samurai@yahoo.com
Sent: Friday, August 26, 10:52 a.m.
Subject: Re: me first...

so tired...
clinging to a cup of coffee.

as uncomfortable as it was,
it was nice to feel you next to me.
even if your body temperature
compares to the center of the sun.

even if i am.

From: le_samurai@yahoo.com

To: chasityrae@gmail.com

Sent: Friday August 26, 11:34 a.m.

Subject: Re: me first...

sorry you're so tired...

yes, it was nice
to wake up with you
by my side...
and then wake up again...
and again...

body heat...
so?
i have CANCER, okay?
jeez...

From: chasityrae@gmail.com

To: le_samurai@yahoo.com

Sent: Friday, August 26, 3:53 p.m.

Subject: Re: me first...

body heat?
it doesn't come close
to describing how
warm you were last night!

and the cancer excuse...
doesn't work with me, buddy.

I'm glad it will be winter soon.
my own human furnace.

From: le_samurai@yahoo.com
To: chasityrae@gmail.com
Sent: Friday, August 26, 4:28 p.m.
Subject: hmmmm

maybe we should go
to your house for a nap?
do you know what a "nooner" is?
hmmmmiwonder...

chapter twenty-one

secret heart

You do stupid things when someone you love has cancer. Like Google the disease and the outcome. You research treatment options and life expectancies. You look at pictures of individuals fighting the same cancer, of receiving chemo, of tumors and surgeries. You read about symptoms and side effects. You read about celebrities like Katie Couric and wonder if you could call her at home. Ask her how she did it. How did she care for her husband during cancer?

I remember—maybe not the exact date, but I remember the moment. I remember going to a bookstore, alone. I did it sometimes when I needed to clear my head. I told Anthony I was going shopping or meeting a friend. I just went to the bookstore. As a means to escape, I'd pick up romance or sci-fi books, or any other kind of novel I would never normally buy, and get lost in the characters. I'd spend hours reading first chapters.

even if i am.

That day I sat on the floor of the health section surrounded by books on colon cancer: books I never read, in a section of the bookstore I never explored. I skimmed through dozens of newly revised paperbacks, looking for a positive sign, a clear end to the disease, and an answer to everything that was happening to us. Printed books held more weight than the online garbage I had been reading. I looked, relentlessly, at book after book, page after page. I found nothing encouraging. Read only grim statistics and outcomes, numbers and facts and testimonials.

Even with apparent warning signs typed out in bold font, I ignored the facts and focused on what I knew. Our story was about love, not cancer. Cancer was someone else's story, like Katie Couric. I put the dismal books back on the shelf and smiled wide. Our love was unique, even miraculous. Our love could cure cancer, even if there was only an eight percent chance of survival.

...

From: le_samurai@yahoo.com
To: chasityrae@gmail.com
Sent: Tuesday, August 30, 3:05 p.m.
Subject: you're right...

i should have written

but i called,

and wrote two texts...
and an e-mail after that
seemed to be a little obsessive...

besides, you're looking way too sexy today
for me to deny a modest request...
i think it's the happiness and excitement
of you producing, working hard,
that's making you stand straight,
and fucking shine...

reminds me a little of when we first met...
oh god, this is turning into
another hallmark card isn't it???

this is the second day
i've been off my chemo,
and i can feel the difference...
a reminder of what things
used to feel like...
weird.
but very, very good...
and my radiologist said
i am almost one third
of the way through my treatments...
i've done nine, and there are 28 in all...
crazy, right?

You were strong in spite of chemo and radiation, regardless of the occasional side effects. Your doctor prescribed pills, a rainbow of "just in case" options. I called them: "puke pills" to deal with nausea, "poop pills" to deal with diarrhea, "sleepy pills" for sleeping, and "yucky pills" for chemo. You know, clever names. We had backup pills in both cars, at my house, at yours, and at work. We were prepared to kick any side effect. And we did. We managed. Job well done.

...

From: chasityrae@gmail.com
To: le_samurai@yahoo.com
Sent: Friday, September 2, 6:39 p.m.
Subject: aw crap!

I heard a rumor that you and I are dating?
no seriously, a co-worker said
he heard a rumor that we are dating...
(he guessed you, or Zach).

I laughed and said nothing.

From: le_samurai@yahoo.com

To: chasityrae@gmail.com

Sent: Friday, September 2, 6:54 p.m.

Subject: Re: aw crap!

hmmmm... dating, eh?
well, let's see...
next time you're asked (or i am)
let's have some other options available:

1. "no, we don't go on dates, we just have sex..."
2. "dating? oh no, he's just my rebound..."
3. "no comment."
4. "we are 2 mature 2 be 4 gotten"
5. "is that what you heard? well, i heard you're retarded. care to comment?"

the last one is my favorite so far...
maybe you have some ideas?

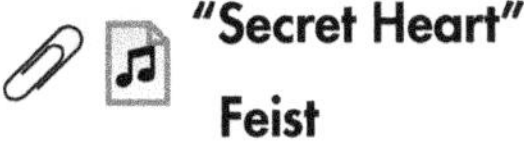
"Secret Heart"
Feist

...

I'm not sure who thought it was the best idea. Either way, we agreed. We'd keep our relationship secret until you were healthy. You didn't want to be introduced to family and friends as, “My boyfriend with cancer.” I don’t blame you. I certainly didn’t want my grandma or dad to worry about me. I already had them concerned when I ended a five-year relationship and began living on my own. They were fearful I was making poor choices with my life. This would surely top their poor-choice list. And what if you got really sick? Or appeared sick? Or lost your hair? What would I tell them then? It seemed appropriate to keep our relationship secret. I’m not mad at you for this necessity. It made sense. In fact, I think it was my idea. Surely I wanted to tell everyone that I met someone, found true love. I wanted to share the very secret I had to conceal—my secret heart. But we put it off, agreeing, “One step at a time.”

The end of chemo was in sight. Next, we needed to get through surgery.

chapter twenty-two

rainy day

Counting down the days to surgery was like waiting for a vacation to Hawaii. I x'ed days off the calendar as you packed our suitcase. Hope had us high with anticipation. Though, with so much emotion came the inevitable roller-coaster ride of love fests and fights. Anxiety about a looming surgery led to crappy behavior—from both of us.

"What should I cook for dinner?" I asked one night.

"Um, eggs sound good?"

"Breakfast for dinner, eh?"

"Sounds yummy. Babe, mind if I lie down? I'm not feeling great."

I thought I could be helpful, cook dinner and let you get some rest. I went to the kitchen, pulled out the frying pan, eggs and sausages. As the eggs cooked I sprinkled cheese on top. I never paid much attention to the details of cooking. It was a must-do task, and always tedious. My mind wandered to someday in the future, when "not feeling great" meant a cold or a headache. I thought of kissing you on our wedding day. I could see us summering in Maine with your family, splashing in the lake. I left the plastic spatula leaning on the frying pan's edge, eggs bubbling, sausages browning and went to check on you. Babe, you looked so comfortable, warm and cozy. I wanted to jump in and snuggle. Instead I let you rest and went back to the stove. I grabbed the plastic spatula. Heat stung my fingers, and the plastic melted into my palm.

I threw the utensil across the room, shrieking in pain.

You came running to my aid.

"Never mind," I snapped. "I'm fine." I immediately pulled away then turned my back. I soaked my hand in cold water, removing the melted plastic from my palm. After cooling the burn, I hurried to the medicine cabinet and applied salve.

I looked for you in the bedroom. You were sitting on the bed, clearly upset. "Are you feeling better?" I said, calm.

"No." You forced the word out between your teeth.

"Are you mad at me?"

"Yes."

"Why?"

"'Cause you told me to leave you alone."

"No I didn't."

"Yes. You did. Maybe not those exact words, but I felt like you didn't need me."

"I didn't. I'm fine. It's just a small burn." I quieted my voice. I wanted the conversation to head back to us in love.

"But I could've helped," you snapped.

"How?"

"I don't know, comforted you or something."

"It's just a burn."

"But I wanted to help! The spatula melted into your hand."

"Don't be an asshole."

"Don't push me away when you're hurt. I can still take care of you. I'm not helpless." You were grasping for control of the situation; so was I.

"I never said you were."

"But that's how I felt." You turned your head away from me.

"I'm sorry. It's just a stupid burn. Big deal."

Isn't it funny how a conversation could just slip away from us, babe? How a long, awkward silence could fill the room. I stared at my burnt palm, then reached for your shoulder to comfort you.

"I'm not hungry," you said breaking the quiet.

"What?"

"I said I'm not hungry."

"Why?"

"'Cause, I'm not."

"But you haven't eaten anything." I could hear my voice rise.

"So?"

"Anthony."

"I'm feeling nauseated, okay? I just took my puke pills."

"Why didn't you say something?"

"'Cause you're hurt."

"Oh my God, it's just a small burn."

"I'm going home. I feel nauseated and the smell of your eggs is going to make me throw up."

"You've got to be kidding me." I shook my head. "Fine. Go."

It was my fault. I pushed you away. My burn was so minor. I wanted you to rest and then join me for dinner, not care for my hand. You weren't feeling good. I'm sorry, Anthony. I was stressing. With surgery around the corner, side effects, and meeting your mom, I had a lot to deal with. I was pretending everything was fine between us—not even okay, but extraordinary. And when things weren't extraordinary between us, I took it out on you. It was foolish, but I wanted to be strong, not struggling with uncertainty.

I ate my eggs alone that night. Then, led by regret, I e-mailed you.

From: chasityrae@gmail.com
To: le_samurai@yahoo.com
Sent: Saturday, September 10, 11:30 p.m.
Subject: when did it become so difficult?

we have gone too far into the serious side,
that we keep losing track.
damnit, let's have fun already,
stop focusing on the problems, on cancer
and enjoy the moments we spend together...

because if this relationship isn't fun,
then what are we doing?

I knew you were mad at me, but somehow this was different. I screwed up. You made sure I knew; you didn't e-mail back.

...

The smell of rain humidified the air. I hit snooze twice, three times. I'm convinced rain in Los Angeles should be considered a snow day, a break from routine, from working hard, and a day to stay under the blankets. Even Gladys didn't want to undo the tight ball of her sleeping body.

Contemplating a fourth snooze, I heard a knock on the door. Doubtful it was my house, I rolled over. Another knock disturbed the chilled room. What the hell do the neighbors want at eight in the morning? I dragged myself out from the depths of my comforter and headed to the door. Gladys didn't budge.

Soaking from the rain, bright yellow sunflowers glowed just under your chin. Babe, I was shocked to see you. Apprehension had me concerned what I was wearing; my polar bear pants that I've had since high school and a sleeveless t-shirt from a previous decade. Nope. Not sexy at all. I brushed the front of my sleeveless to straighten the wrinkles, then opened the screen door.

"I didn't know you were coming." I'm an idiot.

You didn't say a word, just stood there in the rain, looking all cute and cuddly and sweet.

"Anthony, I'm sor—"

"I love you more." You interrupted. There was no time for apologies; we were too busy taking off wet clothes and polar bear pants.

"Thank you for the flowers…"

You kissed the back of my head as we spooned.

"I'm sorry I didn't eat your eggs."

…

From: le_samurai@yahoo.com
To: chasityrae@gmail.com
Sent: Monday, September 12, 10:20 a.m.
Subject: rainy day

rainy day at work…
i think everyone here
is having the same thought we had
when we were on your bed
(stay home and cuddle).

it felt wonderful bringing you flowers,
being a boy, and you being a girl…
mmmmm…

thinking of all the things

we could be doing in your bed...
reading, napping, loving,
glayds jumping up to get
in the middle of the two of us,

making oatmeal and coffee,
drinking hot tea in sweaters,
getting under your covers
and taking everything off...

fuck!
it should rain more often...
and what the hell are we doing here?

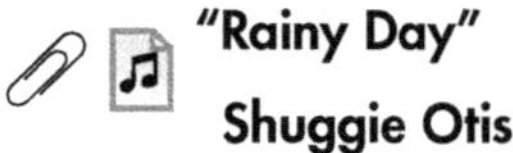
"Rainy Day"
Shuggie Otis

Shuggie Otis gave me the same giddy reaction that I felt after reading your first-ever e-mail. You know, I'm not sure when a honeymoon phase starts or ends. You hear stories about meeting "the one." The characters comically extract themselves from problems and get on with their destinies. In real life, I didn't know if I was pursuing the right path or not, or how it would all work out—I could only hope that this ugly reality was part of attaining a fat, fulfilling love. This seemed to be the right time in our lives for falling in love, for paying off student loans, building credit, and house hunting. The time when we hoped for an engagement, considered having children—in short, when we should start making a future based on our love.

Yet, we worried about cancer. Babe, we'd get so caught up in coping, filling our days with tasks and to-dos, getting bogged down in circumstances, feeling angry at your diagnosis, treatments, and surgery. The worst part… Anthony, you'd be mad at me if I told you this sooner, but the worst part was that I'd get so caught up in it that I'd forget you loved me. I know it seems silly. How could someone forget they're loved? I don't know. But, I did sometimes.

chapter twenty-three

be mine

Friday, October 21
the first post.

this could be the beginning, or possibly the end.

posted by Anthony Glass at 9:54 a.m.

This was the first post to your blog. It was such a simple sentence. I didn't understand what you were going through, I certainly tried, but I didn't. I could only tell from an outside perspective the effects cancer had on you. Your blog described your cancer better than anyone could. It was a brilliant idea, the perfect outlet. A place for you to freely write out your tears. You told me you felt better for having expressed yourself, rather than trying to shunt your self-expression into unsatisfying conversations with friends and family. On your blog, you swore, threatened and raged about cancer. The world could read your clinical process chart on coping: at first anguish and confusion. Next anger and resolution, then comedy, tragedy, hope and despair. It was all there. If anyone wanted to know how you were doing, all we had to do was click and read.

Friday, October 22
(this was written on the 18th)

it wasn't a long day, per se
but it's getting late,
and a long pull from a tall bottle of beer
slows my mind enough that i can discard the to-do lists.
what was done and what was forgotten,
and just let myself appreciate the day
for what it was and what it wasn't.

so often i am on the verge of easing,
but the small splinters jab just enough.

is it possible to be organized and together
without being a complete tightass?
working on it.
answers pending.
doctors.
assistants.
bureaucracy.
forms.

be mine

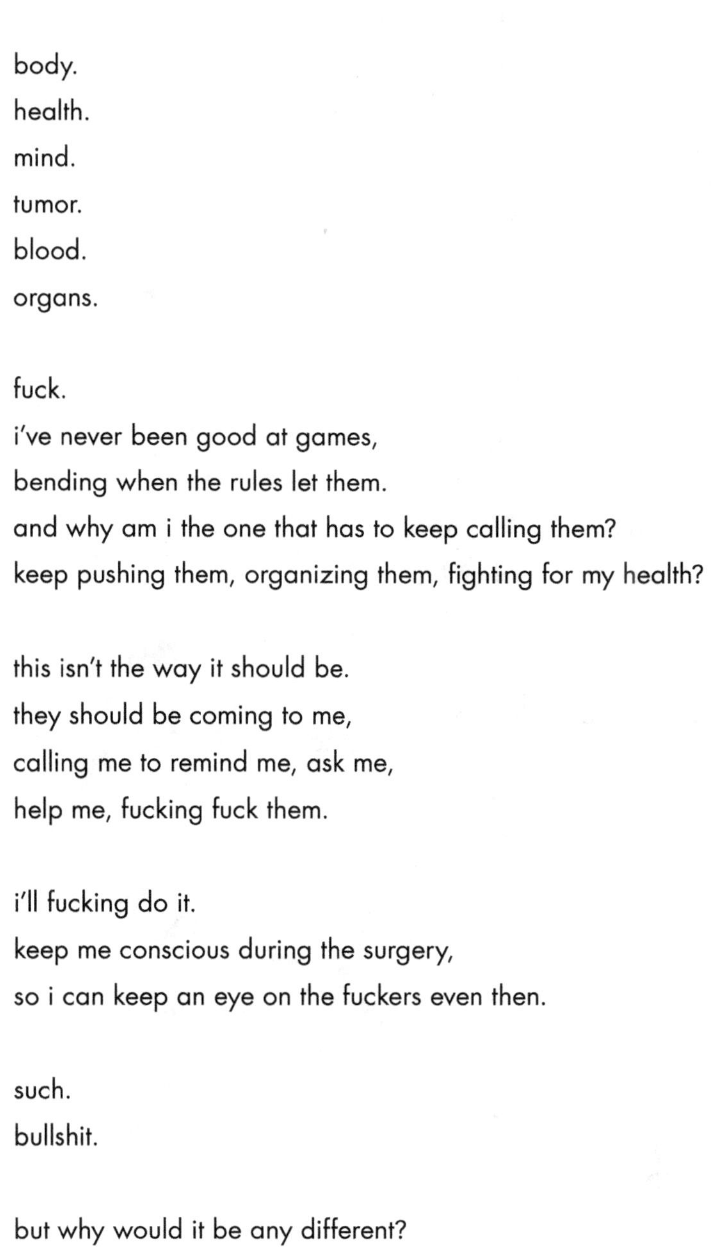

rules.

body.
health.
mind.
tumor.
blood.
organs.

fuck.
i've never been good at games,
bending when the rules let them.
and why am i the one that has to keep calling them?
keep pushing them, organizing them, fighting for my health?

this isn't the way it should be.
they should be coming to me,
calling me to remind me, ask me,
help me, fucking fuck them.

i'll fucking do it.
keep me conscious during the surgery,
so i can keep an eye on the fuckers even then.

such.
bullshit.

but why would it be any different?

cancer didn't make me grow wings out of my back.
why would it make the health care system
suddenly efficient and simple?

alright.
enough rant.

posted by Anthony Glass at 9:54 a.m.

...

From: chasityrae@gmail.com
To: le_samurai@yahoo.com
Sent: Tuesday, October 18, 10:12 a.m.
Subject: a blog

I read your blog this morning...
it is so incredibly
intimate
sincere
sweet
tender
and
heartfelt.

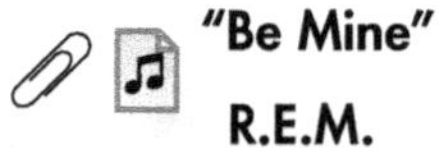
"Be Mine"
R.E.M.

Anthony, reading your words, I wanted to smother you with kisses and ask you to never leave me. I wanted to marry you right then and have a dozen children starting that afternoon. I did. I wanted to. I wanted to *comb the tar out of your feathers; pluck the thorns out of your feet.* I wanted to love you like a revolution, and you to love me equally. *If you made me your religion, I'd give you all you need. I'd be the drawing of your breath, the cup if you should bleed. I'd be the lights that guide you inland. You and me.*

I wanted to find you right then. To rub your face, look you in the eyes and tell you just how much I love you. I wished I could have done more to help—wished I could take away your pain. I wished I was the one with cancer. I know, I know. But, I did. I wished I were the one fighting. I loved you so much; I was scared to tell you how much. Instead, I told you, "Your blog is beautiful. It helps us understand."

chapter twenty-four

naked as we came

Every part of us thought about, stressed about, and argued about cancer. There was a lot to plan, a lot going on, making the circumstances delicate. The closer to surgery and the more medications you took, our sex became, well, awkward. It was awkward, right? I don't know how someone fights about sex; maybe all couples fight about sex, but during sex? We managed to find a motive.

Even now, it hurts in new and varied ways. Maybe you felt defeated and needed someone to blame. I'd like to think it was your belly full of chemo, and not my fault. I wasn't in the mood for sex that night. You pushed me at my worst, sometimes. I'm not blaming you. Okay, maybe a little, but I had a hundred things on my mind. Work was busy as ever. I hadn't called my family in weeks. We had another big CAT scan that afternoon, a thousand things were going through my mind, but you persisted, pushed. "No and no." It didn't help that I said it through a giggle as you kissed my neck.

even if i am.

You knew how to turn my no's into yes's. Your lips on my skin were a weakness. We kissed as my legs wrapped around you like twine. Then it happened. My mind shifted back to the thoughts stirring inside.

"Ouch. Sorry, but you're pulling my hair."

Instantly you struggled. "Would you focus on me?"

"I am. But, my hair was under..." You're right. I wasn't focusing on you. I couldn't get in the mood no matter where you kissed. I tried. I did, I swear. But a million little thoughts got in the way.

"This is too much work." I knew that tone. Irritated, you rolled off of me. "You make me jump through hoops to get you in the mood. And you smell funny. Did you even shower today?"

"Okay, now you're just being a jerk. Did I shower today? Asshole."

I got up from the bed and put my shirt on as you looked for your pants, complaining about our sex life. Listing all the things I'd done wrong until that point. I equal parts loved you and couldn't stand you.

...

From: chasityrae@gmail.com
To: le_samurai@yahoo.com
Sent: Wednesday, October 26, 11:46 a.m.
Subject: hurt

last night's conversation hurt, bad...
and it wasn't so much what you said,
it hurt because I think it's not me you love,
but merely the idea of me you love.

Since the day we started this relationship you have tried to modify me into a version of someone you preferred. Contacts over glasses, express more, don't flirt too much, don't hang out with. After last night's conversation, I realized that I can NEVER be the girl you're wanting me to be. I have flaws and faults that define who I am, things you will love and hate; more importantly, things that I cannot or do not want to change.

Last night I felt as if you had blamed me for our fighting, and then if blaming me wasn't enough, you began to list things wrong with me sexually. I don't express myself, I don't tell you how I like it, or what turns me on, I push and pull, I don't pay enough attention, I never initiate... I smell?

NEVER have I felt this insecure about my actions.

even if i am.

NEVER have I felt uncomfortable in my own skin.
NEVER have I second guessed my self-worth, who I am, or what fucking shoes am I gonna wear...

this is not me, and it feels gross.

I can't keep hurting like this.
I can't keep questioning myself and my actions.

Maybe we are putting too much on this relationship because we are so emotionally invested. Maybe we both desperately want that perfect relationship and commitment, and maybe, just maybe, neither of us are willing to admit that "we" aren't the right match.

I wish I knew the answers,
I wish I could be the girl you needed me to be.
I wish for a lot of things...
but I don't wish to feel like this anymore.

From: le_samurai@yahoo.com
To: chasityrae@gmail.com
Sent: Wednesday, October 26, 2:23 p.m.
Subject: Re: hurt

i love you.*

*although a simple statement, it seems there are a number of ways this can be interpreted, distorted, feared, and even mutilated. my love for you is simple. it does not come with the expectations that you are "the one," with a prescribed order of physical and personality traits you must be trained to have in order to fulfill this persona. that's bullshit. my love for you is simple. it is for you.

we have many differences, basic things about us.
at times it seems they will be our undoing.
times like these.

the thought of it makes me sick,
but what are we doing?
i can't believe it was only yesterday
that you were here in my office,
our arms wrapped around each other,
and i felt like i was going to jump out of my body
just to get a little bit closer to you.
and here we are?

i understand what you feel
when you say you're tired,
because it's fucking exhausting.

all morning i've been writing this,
and my feelings are all over the place.
but beneath it all, i can't imagine

even if i am.

not being with you, and giving up.
i know you're feeling right now
that perhaps that's the best thing,
and maybe you're right.
i really don't know.

i do recognize that i am
a hippopotamus trying to do ballet
when it comes to being tactful or delicate,
but if you smell funny,
i want to fucking tell you. that's intimacy.
tell me my dick is crooked. it is.

too much writing.
too much thinking.
sending this now because it's taken too long,
and i know you're waiting for it.

...

I blame Snow White. Yep, Snow White. She made love seem easy. She wished in a well for the one she loved to find her; and then there he was, a dashing prince galloping in on a white horse. They hardly exchanged two words. I think: Just wait, honey. Just wait until you fight over chores, awkward sex, meeting parents or cancer. Snow White, you know nothing about love.

Yet, I listened. I believed in once-upon-a-times and happily-ever-afters. Because of Snow White I got my heart broken. Over and over. I kept thinking, he's coming, my happily-ever-after. Just wish into the goddamn well. I waited for him. I waited for him at a seventh grade dance, then again in homeroom, in college studying art, at the bar sipping a PBR, the grocery store buying two-ply toilet paper... I eventually found him—three times, actually. The truth was disappointing, yet I refused to give up on the fairytale.

"I'm not done loving you," I e-mailed back.

...

From: le_samurai@yahoo.com
To: chasityrae@gmail.com
Sent: Thursday, October 27, 10:59 a.m.
Subject: never be done

let's have dinner
just the two of us tonight.
well, three of us if you count gladys...

do you want to help me come up with
questions to ask the surgeon tomorrow?
some possibilities:
will anthony be as much of an asshole

after surgery as he is right now?
think about it.

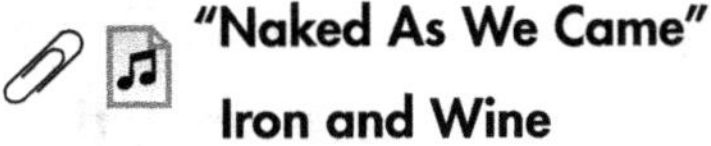

"Naked As We Came"
Iron and Wine

chapter twenty-five

in the round

From: le_samurai@yahoo.com

To: friends

Sent: Friday, October 28, 3:27 p.m.

Subject: web+log=blog!

my dear friends and family,
if you are receiving this e-mail
it means that you are pretty frickin' special,
and in an effort to stay close with each of you
over the next weeks and months,
i have started a blog to post
the latest news/events/thoughts/images,
so that if you're ever wondering,
you have someplace to go
to see/read/feel the latest.

http://anthonyglass.blogspot.com

love to all.

a.

Thursday, October 27
and all of a sudden

getting ready to meet with my surgeon this afternoon,
writing my list of questions to ask him... kind of slow going...
question #1: "how much is this going to suck?"
question #2: "how long is this going to suck for?"

this month has flown by,
and as eager as i was for the surgery to arrive,
it's two weeks away, and i can't help but feel
like that's suddenly much closer than i thought.

as a follow-up to the chemo and radiation therapy,
two days ago i had to go in to get an imaging scan
of my abdomen to see how my insides are looking.
as is standard practice, i had to down two liters
of barium contrast (with a delightful citrus flavor).
it was disgusting, and i'm quite sure if i ever need
to vomit on cue in the future, i'll have plenty of motivation.

still facing the obstacles of blue cross.
writing my appeal to get my surgeon Dr. Beart covered*
feels something like writing a personal statement

to get into a college i know will never accept me.
but maybe if i write something so absolutely brilliant...
right.

*quality costs money.

posted by Anthony Glass at 9:54 a.m.

From: le_samurai@yahoo.com
To: chasityrae@gmail.com
Sent: Friday, October 28, 2:59 p.m.
Subject: cuddle

after spending the whole morning
putting my blog together
and sending out the e-mail,
i find myself finally getting into work...
i guess it's a good thing
since i have to leave before three
to meet my surgeon.

i think you have a lot of reasons
for coming down to cuddle
and should use any one of them to do so.
i will look forward to it.

just in case i didn't send it before,
here it is again...

even if i am.

this morning was beautiful,
come visit me soon.

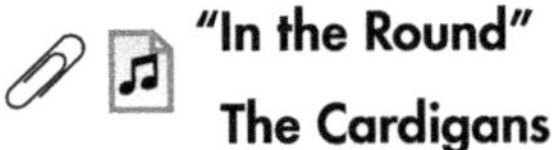

From: chasityrae@gmail.com
To: le_samurai@yahoo.com
Sent: Friday, October 28, 3:31 a.m.
Subject: Re: cuddle

maybe it's the cold weather
or that my tummy hurts
or that you're leaving for the day
or that you are meeting with your surgeon
or that I'm not going with

whatever it is...
I miss you.

...

Your family became long-distance caregivers. Your mother gave emotional, spiritual support and dietary advice during each call; stepfather coordinated medical services via telephone. Your brothers distracted you with football and reminisced about childhood. I was thankful when your stepfather decided to fly in from D.C. for two days to meet your surgeon, Dr. Beart, for a second opinion. The first was a general HMO surgeon who didn't seem skilled enough for such a complex and detailed surgery. He had never even worked on a colon. We looked for and found the best possible colon cancer specialist in Los Angeles. Surely your stepfather, being a doctor himself, would have questions and concerns that were more valid than my petty worries.

We never planned an introduction. I'd meet your stepfather when there was time to visit, not between doctor appointments.

...

I'm a sucker for dance movies—*Footloose*, *Dirty Dancing*, *Step Up 2: The Streets*, it doesn't matter. I cry. Flashdance nearly hospitalized me. So unless I'm feeling pathetic enough to seek out a serious cathartic moment, I avoid dance movies.

Hope. That's what gets me, every time. The basic idea of hope, the obstacle to overcome, the music chosen to extract tears—I'm an absolute sucker. "Just let her dance! One. More. Time." I scream at the television. Dance movies are my kryptonite (long pause for dramatic effect) until now (longer pause). There is something out there far worse than dance movies. Just reading a show description makes me sob. Medical dramas. There's no form of entertainment more littered with hope than the medical drama. Hope that they save the old man from heart failure, hope that the woman can conceive after the accident, hope that the child doesn't lose a limb after the near-fatal infection. Hope that his surgery removes the tumor…

Sunday, October 30
it's all happening…

the weekend has expired,
left itself in small pieces
in forgotten places
(it is sunday night, after all).

picking them up, folding them neatly,
and putting them away
(monday comes better that way).

the best news in recent memory came thursday afternoon,
when meeting with my surgeon
for my post-therapy, pre-surgery consult.
he told me the tumor
had responded very well to the radiation and chemo,
and had dramatically reduced in size
allowing for a much smaller section
to be removed when i have surgery november 16th.

i was, however, in mid-exam when i received the news,
and tempered my joy until the anal-scope was removed
and my ass was lowered from the mechanized exam table

that had it perched five feet high in the air.

needless to say,
once i was back on my feet
i was ecstatic.

went to see charlie kaufman at the writers' guild,
and was reminded of so many things,
so many good things.

halloween party at a house
i don't live in anymore.
everyone dressed up as someone else.
but there were some familiar faces,
and it was fun, especially the part when i went home,
quiet home.
peaceful home.

feel like a squirrel nesting in here,
trying to get everything ready
with winter fast approaching.
counting my acorns.

good news:
happiness is available for all
in the form of $12 slippers from target.

even if i am.

they might've changed my life.

posted by Anthony Glass at 10:45 p.m.

chapter twenty-six

mexico

From: le_samurai@yahoo.com

To: chasityrae@gmail.com

Sent: Wednesday, November 2, 10:08 a.m.

Subject: on the road

this is a sweet song,
a familiar voice.
something that makes me
want to pack up the car
and drive south...

yes, i know...
when will that be us?
driving on the mexican coast
on the road to ensenada.

maybe we'll go somewhere for christmas or new year's.

even if i am.

would mexico be fun for that?
feels like it.

i'm so curious to see
how i heal from the surgery,
but i'm expecting to be
feeling solid by new year's.
solid.

seems pretty far off though, huh?
sigh.

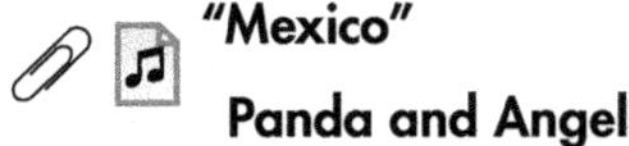

...

A naked man Photoshopped from *Playgirl* with a scary resemblance to you adorned the invitation to celebrate Anthony Day.

Anthony's more than just a sweet piece of ass (and that's good, because the doctors will be removing that piece soon), so join us as we celebrate his better qualities, whatever they may be! Bring your booze, leave your pants!

...

"So explain it to me again slowly, who are York and Julie?"

I can't believe we'd been dating for months already. It took me by surprise that I was getting ready for a party to meet your friends. Besides Zach, I hadn't really met anyone; but I'd heard the stories about drunken-rowdy-night-friends, old roommates, and secret crushes. I knew most of the stories behind the nicknames Antone, Crazy Tony, Thony, and Beautiful Anthony, but I had yet to put a face to the long list of names on the Evite.

York and his girlfriend Julie, the hosts of the party, were first to greet me. You're right. York is a bit intimidating, and his height doesn't help. He towered over me, and bombarded me with the uncomfortable question, "Do you know Anthony's nickname is Glassanova? How do you feel about that?" I didn't even say hello. Instead I laughed nervously as Julie gave you a kiss, greeting you, "Ah, my beautiful Anthony." Julie was mostly sweet, though certainly considered me another of the "Glassanova" girls. You never did tell me about that nickname—then again, we never played the "how many people have you been with" game. It's probably for the best.

Guests began arriving. Zach was one of the first and dating a new blonde who kept me distracted with random conversation. Your good friend Jane flirted with this strange guy named Seth whose annoying voice sounded like a yogi's chant. Jay came with an ex-girlfriend, a rumored tornado.

Former co-workers mingled with current. Ex-girlfriends chatted with friends of friends. A guy smoked on the patio and put too much dip on his chip. A brunette with a low-cut shirt bent over to towel her spilled wine, looking up to see who was admiring.

It was amusing meeting everyone and I think I did well, considering that this party was our coming out. I can't recall a single conversation, only my nervous anticipation and fragments of that night. The girls who actually arrived wearing no pants. Your breath smelled of green tea. The bit of spinach dip smeared on your lower lip as you smiled at me across the kitchen. Even though I wanted to be selfish and have you all to myself, this was your party. You mattered to everyone in the room. Our task was to say a holy hell yes to you. We did it with Jell-O shots, chips, cigarettes, girls missing pants, and drawn-out stories of rowdier days.

When no one was watching we made kissy faces across the room. We drifted close to each other, touching toe to toe, your hand on the small of my back. Just enough touch to reassure.

...

From: le_samurai@yahoo.com
To: chasityrae@gmail.com
Sent: Tuesday, November 8, 9:41 a.m.
Subject: work

mmmmkay...
its almost 10 a.m.
and i haven't done any work.

i have written a new post,
and it feels great
to have gotten it out.
there is therapy online.

but i wanted you to know
that i am very much thinking of you,
and i can't wait to spend the night with you.

jumping into my edits now,
maybe i'll find you there.

Tuesday, November 8
and i am a creature of habit

going to the sidelines,
we always see the game

even if i am.

with a different eye.

can it be that i'm only a week from surgery?
that this is the last week at work?

although part of me smiles at the thought
of not being here day in and day out
and having to drive across town twice a day,
another part feels slightly shaken.

my office,
my edit bay.
my little meditation room.
it is a place of security and comfort.
a personal place, a private hideaway
(yeah, until someone bursts the door open
by mistake thinking it's the stairwell).

and the people.
friendships that have grown out of this place,
and acquaintances, that despite their sincerity
never seem to get beyond these walls.
they will all remain, running in place,
wearing the carpet just a little thinner beneath their feet.

who will be in my bay when i am gone?

it is a strange thing to disconnect yourself

from the routine and system you're accustomed to.
and i am a creature of habit.
morning pb & j.
afternoon walk for coffee.

planning on working from home a few weeks after surgery,
and then coming back to the office in the new year.
i guess that's the new routine.
the new system.

an interesting holiday season this will be.

posted by Anthony Glass at 8:39 a.m.

chapter twenty-seven

in the deep

"I've spent the morning on the phone with the hospital and Blue Cross. It looks pretty shitty."

"How shitty?"

"The surgeon is out of my network plans and won't be covered. I'm submitting my appeal to Blue Cross via fax this morning, but it looks like I'll be paying $40,000 out of pocket. Up front? Fuck. Honestly, I kind of expected all of this, so it's not hitting me as a surprise, just more of a disappointment. I should have handled this whole mess earlier rather than waiting until the week of surgery. I thought I had reformed my procrastinating ways… talked to my mom yesterday and she said she was bringing the home equity checkbook. I should call her again before she gets on the plane to prepare her for what's coming."

"I'm so sorry, babe. Is there anything I can do?"

"No. I just need to get this letter out. Dinner with my mom should be fun tonight. Right?"

even if i am.

...

Men worship their mothers. Studying Freud in college convinced me and the rest of the human race of such basics. The Oedipus complex: the desire to possess the parent of the opposite sex. So, it came as no surprise when you raved about your mother. That's what sons do. They hold in high regard. And when you told me your mother was beautiful, I figured every son says that about his mother.

But your mother was absolutely dazzling. Her hair perfectly straight, thick stunning shades of grey. The top half pulled back to reveal her strong features. High cheekbones, powerful eyes, perfect lips, a soft glow off her skin shimmering twenty years younger than her age. She didn't need make-up to show off her beauty. Make-up would have only distracted. I couldn't stop staring at her during dinner. I should have guessed her voice to be persuasive, soothing; she's a therapist who works with children.

I was nervous. I said very little as the two of you talked about health, strength, surgeon, fees, and procedures. You turned boyish in your mother's presence. I tried to interrupt, give my opinion when necessary and seem useful. It came across aggressive. Then I complimented the taste of my pork chop just to say something. You looked at me funny. What? It was my first time meeting her, and it was under unusual circumstances. I wondered how many other girlfriends met your mother.

"Mmm, this pork chop is delicious. Would you like to try a bite?" I actually offered her a bite of my pork chop.

...

From: le_samurai@yahoo.com
To: chasityrae@gmail.com
Sent: Wednesday, November 16, 9:56 a.m.
Subject: and so

it is becoming late in the afternoon,
and the sun is setting lower in the sky,
lower than it should for this time of the day,
but i guess that's the kind of light
and the kind of feeling
this time of year brings.

i know i must be feeling overwhelmed
because all i want to do is fall asleep,
and wake up when everything is as it was
instead of as it is.

at times,
i see this all as a good thing,
as life-saving.
i think about what this could have become
had i gone untreated.

even if i am.

other times,
i can't help but feel frustrated with myself,
for not catching this sooner,
and think about how i could have prevented
everything that's happening right now.

i think about the first incision,
and feel like i will be forever altered,
damaged, changed.

people lose limbs.
lose organs.
lose lives.

i am losing a part of my body.
a bad part.

i need to remember that.
this is a beginning,
not an end.

and you.
are you crying yet, reading this?
i don't know how to describe
the way i feel with/for you right now,
and i know i've thanked you
for being as close and strong
as you've been with me

through this entire fucking mess,
but i don't think you really understand.

after covering the entire emotional gamut
over the past nine months,
i don't quite know how we've landed
in the soft and secure place we're in right now,
but i am so happy that we have.
it feels like we're fulfilling what we both saw
at the very beginning.

christ, is this melodramatic?
okay, i've got a ton to do,
and you just sent me a sweet text…
cuddle.
yes, the thought of it makes me smile.

i will call you soon.
and will see you shortly thereafter.
i love you.

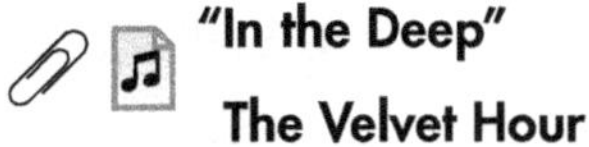

…

I was trying to put on a brave face. This stupid, lame thought kept creeping in, wondering if I'd ever see you again. I wasn't ready to lose you to cancer. The idea was so overwhelming sad. It's just a simple surgery. I tried convincing myself.

Maybe I wasn't your mother's favorite, and maybe I was trying too hard for her to like me, but I was thankful for her presence. "Can I make you some tea?" I asked, because I didn't know what else to do. She was such a great source of relief, and I felt useless.

...

From: le_samurai@yahoo.com
To: friends
Sent: Wednesday, November 16, 2:01 p.m.
Subject: real quick

you're all fucking amazing,
and the support and love i have felt
for the last couple of weeks,
and especially the last couple of days
has quite simply been stunning.
thank you. all.
(especially york and julie for sponsoring saturday night.)

going in tomorrow morning at 9 a.m., surgery at 11 a.m.
and as much as i would love to see you all
while in a delirious, drug-induced state,
i won't be up for visitors until the weekend.
so save your love until then.

and then bring it.
and give me a sponge bath with it...
yum.

below is the link for the hospital/department,
and if you have any questions about my condition
or are planning to come by to visit,
please call chas's cellphone.

http://ccnt.hsc.usc.edu/colorectal

chapter twenty-eight

what sarah said

CUTTING ACROSS A LONELY PATCH OF THE 405 AS FREEWAY traffic steered south, Death Cab for Cutie sang "What Sarah Said." Your mother stared out the passenger seat window. Our thoughts were miles apart but on the same subject: surgery. Sun lit her reflection and cast a mirrored image in the window, as perfect and poised as the original. She was graceful, calm, present. Or at least that's how she appeared. I resented her for it, and resented her self-control.

All the times I thought this whole thing through, I never thought I'd be edgy and panicked on the day of surgery. After all, we planned this like a vacation. I thought I'd be as calm as your mother—or even that our roles would be reversed.

Hours felt like months. Being a passenger lulled me as I focused on the back of your head. I could have counted each hair. I needed someone to shake me before I went mad trying to compose myself. I hated the back seat. The back seat felt like rejection. I needed you to engage in conversation, to distract me, love me. The uncertainty of you having surgery held this tragic punch. Why? I don't know. I've never even used the word colorectal until now.

I did the only thing I could. I searched for God. Everywhere. I looked for key words in the patterned fabric of the back seat. I closed my eyes, squinted as if He might appear when I wasn't looking. I listened for a voice in the hum of traffic. I looked for Him in the SUVs and sedans that passed. I fantasized God (bare chest and crown of thorns) driving a blue Ford pickup, singing along to Bob Dylan, smiling, giving me the thumbs up as we rolled alongside. I looked for Him in every vehicle, even the BMW convertible I knew He'd never drive. I believed. Maybe not in the stories and biblical sense of God, but I believed in the power and love of something greater than good, something greater than us. When I was six I named God. My mother informed me that God "was the grandfather of all people." I had a friend in Kindergarten who called her grandfather Poppy, and she told me she loved him very much. That Christmas, Santa Claus left me a white teddy bear with a red bow. I named him "Poppy," after God. Poppy the Bear watched over me. Even at age six I felt safe with God, and I believed Poppy was my guardian. And this very moment, in the backseat, I prayed to Poppy again for help.

I rolled down the window to breathe Him in. I looked for Poppy in the air. Not a blink, not a breath, not a sigh of relief. I looked for Him on the beam of light through the window. He wasn't sitting on it. I rested my forehead on the back of the driver's seat, collecting my thoughts, praying as I picked at my cuticles.

Your one arm was steering, and the other grabbed my leg and shook it. "Babe, you want to listen to Death Cab with me?" The simple shake took everything I had. I turned my tears to the passing cars—where the hell is that blue Ford?—as you turned up the radio to let me cry in secret.

...

Valet service?

"It makes patients feel comfortable, gives them one less thing to think about," the man in black explained as he opened the car door. I lingered. My eyes fixed on the massive structure. I couldn't define where it began and where it ended. Your hand felt for mine, and drew me forward into the hospital.

We received nametags, badges for parking, and paperwork, and then assembled in the carpeted corner of the waiting room. Plants and fish aquariums, brochures, magazines, even lamps—lest the hospital feel too homey, framing us were an office door marked Admitting and a large window labeled Cashier.

I don't know who was more thankful, you or I, as your mother filled in the blanks, writing names, social security numbers, and previous health issues. Your hand shook in mine. On the wall across from us was the hospital logo, hands opened with palms facing up. Underneath were the words, "We will raise you up on eagle wings." A lump formed in my throat. By the time I read "wings" I could hardly swallow. I didn't know what to say as you squeezed my hand tighter, my knuckles white.

Your mother gave you the pen. You signed your name. She handed over a check from the home equity checkbook. The cashier directed you to level four for anesthesia.

...

When you were six, your mother planned a family hike along the Tacoma River. She packed a picnic lunch with peanut butter and honey sandwiches, carrots and juice boxes. The plan was to hike down to the river, eat lunch, and hike back. Her boys could enjoy the sunny afternoon, investigate animal tracks, and dip their feet in the cool water.

I've heard the story a hundred times, and even seen pictures, but the first time I heard the story was in the holding area before surgery. You seemed to be as frightened as a boy lost in the woods, only this time you were wearing a blue gown, hair net, IV, and blankets. Even so, you stayed amused at your mother's adaptation of the story, and snickered along with her description of being lost with her three boys in the woods. You'd interrupt with details, specifying which brother took the wrong turn. Every time the story is told, the blame gets passed around. Maybe your mother was so relaxed because she worked in a hospital, but in any case, her voice and her expressions remained soft and light.

The nurse came in and asked standard questions; name, birth date, what sort of surgery you were having, your doctor's name, and then someone from the lab came by to draw blood. Your mother continued the lost woods story until the anesthesia put you to sleep.

...

I paced while your mother read. She and I said very little to each other in the waiting room. The air reeked of Purell, burnt coffee, and nervous sweat. I rationed my breath. I stared at my shoes, unlaced them, and then tied them tighter. I read a mystery that didn't make any sense—mostly because I kept losing track of the characters and plotline. I stared at words on a page. The same page. Waiting. Waiting.

Two hours passed. I thought, I need a little help here Poppy. Tell me he's all right. They had free coffee in the waiting room and I loaded up on a little more than healthy. I drank tea and water. The TV entertained itself, an effortless hum, flickering orange light against families waiting. A woman was summoned by a doctor into the hallway for privacy as I scrutinized the clock. Surely we'd be next. Three hours passed. I was driving your mother nuts. I could literally hear her thinking, for God's sake, woman, would you sit down and relax. I waited for the doctor to enter. I stared at the vending machine imagining the taste of each item within. I planned our future, named children. Prayed. Paced. Picked up my book, put it down.

The doctor came in. There was only your mother and I waiting.

"Mrs. Glass?" We both stood. "Anthony is out of surgery, and everything went well, textbook in fact. There were additional lymph nodes that needed to be removed thus taking a bit longer, but we're confident we removed the existing tumor…"

chapter twenty-nine

EEE. EEE. EEE.

From: chasityrae@gmail.com
To: friends
Sent: Thursday, November 17, 2:42 p.m.
Subject: anthony update

Hello Everyone!

I know you're anxiously awaiting an update, so I'll get right to it. Anthony is doing GREAT!

So good in fact that this morning—yes, I said THIS very morning, only twelve hours after his surgery—he got out of bed and walked down the hallway. An accomplishment he is quite proud of. This of course was only after the sponge bath from the cute nurse (no joke about the cute nurse, not a fantasy. I think it helped boost his motivation, either that or the morphine). His spirits are high (again it might be the drugs).

But, seriously though, he is doing REALLY well!

As for the medical side of things, they are running many tests, results that we will not know for days or weeks. We did have a brief chat with the surgeon who gave us a lot of optimism and said the surgery itself was a "textbook" procedure.

I'll let you know how he is feeling, and will try to give you an update each day. As for now, he should be ready for visitors next Saturday and Sunday.

I want to thank everyone for their love and support. You guys have no idea how much it means to him! I can never thank you enough...

THANKS, again,

Chas

I called it the "shitty shift." Work eight to ten hours, then drive straight to the hospital for dinner. I'd arrive and barely get a kiss before your mother updated me on the day's progress. "He kept rotating his feet and ankles and moving his legs, even with the massaging socks on. The nurse already emptied his catheter for the night, though he ate at least four of the little plastic pitchers of ice. So they might need to change it again."

You shrugged and said, “Num,” your smile still greeting me.

“He said his mouth feels like cotton and his throat is sore. Other than that he feels good. He’s stable now and due to be moved to a private room tomorrow morning. Also the nurse explained the morphine pump. He can self-administer the medication up to five times an hour by pressing the button, but not closer than ten minute intervals. He pressed it five times the first hour. The second hour only about every thirty minutes…”

Your mother’s voice was fidgety from the caffeine consumed throughout the day. She pushed you physically and was pleased with her persistence. “You should’ve seen him…” It was merely the first day and already I had missed so much. I hated it. “He practically ran down the hall…” You were smiling at her and I could feel my skin burning slightly as I smiled. I think you were on to me because you give me that look, the play-nice look.

After her fully detailed progress from your day she departed to her hotel for a comfortable night’s rest. By the time I arrived you were tired of talking about health and exercise and what you ate, crabby from being pushed to your limits, and physically exhausted.

“Hey you.”

“I miss you.”

“I missed you more.” I kissed your soft eyebrow and nestled nose to nose. “How you feeling?”

“I’ll give you a hundred bucks to talk about anything else.”

"I've got some work gossip?"

"Perfect..."

You were asleep twenty minutes into the conversation.

...

I brought blankets and a pillow from home, and settled into my recliner sleeper. There were constant intrusions throughout the night. Blood pressure checks. Blood draws. Flowers delivered at one o'clock. No joke, 1:00 a.m. There were bathroom walks. New IVs. Machines that thumped to heartbeats with monitors attached and ones that administered medications. Beeping machines. Breathing machines. There were weird fluids draining from your sides collecting in small, clear "grenades" that needed draining. Catheters. Random moans and groans of patients down the hallway.

Your mother arrived at six o'clock, refreshed with coffee. Perfectly showered, blushed cheeks, brushed teeth, pressed button-down shirt. She raved about the pillow-top on the hotel bed. If daggers could fire out my eyes they would have pierced her back, right where mine was hurting from the plastic recliner chair.

"Did you go for your morning walk yet?" She eyed me. "Did you walk?"

Seriously, I wanted daggers.

"No, Mama, we just finished breakfast," you said.

EEE. EEE. EEE.

I was starting to really dislike your mother. I scurried off to work puffy-eyed, foul-breathed, and crabby with a backache. The shitty shift.

. . .

From: chasityrae@gmail.com
To: friends
Sent: Friday, November 18, 1:33 p.m.
Subject: sent from work

ANTHONY PASSED GAS!
(He is totally gonna kill me for e-mailing this.)

That's right! Anthony passed gas yesterday, and hopefully more today, which means he starts drinking liquids! Quite the celebration here. YIPPEE! He might be lucky enough to get some Jell-O later tonight. His words: "I could tear the shit out of some Jell-O right now." He is up and walking (four times yesterday) and sitting up in a chair (more activities to celebrate). His energy is high. He's sleeping well, making jokes, typical Anthony.

We have heard only great news from the doctors. The biggest news, which I am sure you are all waiting to hear, is that it looks as though surgery has removed all the cancer present. Of course they are running more tests, and he still has some follow-up therapy, but he is on the road to recovery, and his doctors are very optimistic of the outcome.

So everyone smile, relax, and give Anthony a big kiss when you come to visit him on Saturday or Sunday. Hell, maybe you'll even go for a walk with him down the hall. Again, he is thankful for the e-mails, phone calls, flowers, love and support. He is looking forward to seeing you all this weekend. Visiting hours are anytime. He's generally up by 5 a.m. and asleep by 9 p.m. (naps not included).

See you then!

...

Your mother and I passed notes as we switched shifts.

> *They are hearing all sorts of rumblings inside his intestine. That's great news. Sometime during the afternoon, someone came from respiratory therapy to check his oxygen levels. They left the little blue breathing apparatus, and told him to use it every hour (taking ten breaths, and expelling them). He tends to cough, and it helped immensely for me to rub his tummy and slightly apply pressure. It is very important he does this to prevent mucus from building in his throat and lungs, which will keep him from getting pneumonia. Make sure he does it in the morning when he*

wakes up. There is more Jell-O in the kitchen fridge if he gets hungry. Love, Mom

Before bed he ate some clear soup, Jell-O and a little tea for breakfast. He slept throughout the night. We coughed, blew through plastic machines, and rubbed bellies. Love, Chas

EEE. EEE. EEE. EEE. My swollen eyes caught sight of an IV drip blinking red. I sat up. It was still dark. I fumbled for the lights, molested walls. Trying to stay quiet, I kicked your edge of the bed by accident.

"Shit."

"What time is it?"

"Sorry."

"Do you hear that beeping sound?" you whispered loud.

"Close your eyes, I'm turning on the lights." Half asleep, half awake, I went to find the nurse. She followed me to your room and performed her routine check of machines then left. I lay down. EEE. EEE. EEE. EEE. the beeping continued. I rubbed the walls, kicked the bed again.

"I still hear the beeping?"

"Fuckinghell. I got it. Close your eyes, I'm turning the lights on again."

I frantically looked for the same nurse.

"Excuse me," I said, tapping her shoulder, "the machine is still beeping."

"No, I just checked it. Everything is fine." She walked away.

"I swear to God, lady, the machine keeps beeping. It's what, three a.m.? I'm not making this shit up at three a.m.," I said to the back of her head. Admittedly it was aggressive, but I didn't have the patience.

She marched into your room to prove me wrong. Sure enough, the IV battery needed to be changed. "Ah-*ha*," I said, pointing a finger at her and nodding, waited for her to tell me I was in fact right. I was proud of myself. At last, four days into recovery and I was needed on the shitty shift! I started drafting your mother a letter right then. Finally, I had something worth reporting.

...

Your friend Charlie was the first visitor. If I had met him before I didn't remember. He talked incessantly, was filled with impromptu hospital tales, joked about his motorcycle accidents, broken bones, and split leg. Almost everyone has a crazy uncle who takes them to their first R-rated movie and buys them a beer or a porn mag—and that guy would be Charlie. He was hilarious. He brought romance novels with Fabio on their covers, and puzzles with flying dragons and unicorns as get-well presents.

York, Julie, and friend after friend filed in for comfort and a hug. Bill and Sam arrived, all people I had e-mailed, but couldn't put a face to until now. From the minute visiting hours started until a half past its end, your little room filled with friends, flower arrangements, wacky get well presents and the occasional nurse. The conversation broke its flow only so we could sing "Happy Birthday" to Jay as loud as we could over a cell phone, unashamed of our horrible rendition.

You were our kitchen table, a place for us to rest our elbows on, a place to talk, and share. You held your wound to laugh, and sat upright to give advice to friends complaining about a boyfriend or boss or life. I hadn't seen you smile like that in a long while.

...

From: stepfather
To: chasityrae@gmail.com
Sent: Tuesday, November 18, 5:08 a.m.
Subject: Re: sent from work

Hi, Chas. Thanks for the news. I was dying to hear something, and your e-mail came just before I started back from Italy—sixteen hour trek, with ten hours fighting headwinds over the Atlantic. I am a bit short of sleep the last few days, but probably so are you, with work in the day and being with Anthony at night. He spoke of you a lot during my last visit to see the doctors. So sorry we did not meet. May I say, it's very simple: If Anthony loves you, then so do I.

I am home in Arlington now, but the same e-mail address. I will be most appreciative of any updates you have. On returning I got more details from his mother's e-mail from the business office. I will try the phone now. I will also send some news to the extended family. If you can, in fact, give me daily bulletins. It would be a wonderful gift. Actually, your being there with Anthony is already a wonderful gift.

Well, I'm a bit grogged so will sign off for now. Give Anthony a hug for me. I hope he will give you a hug, for me.

...

I don't know what you thought it would look like, but my mind imagined it gross, crusty, bloody. One eye opened, one closed, I squinted. If it weren't for the doctors complimenting the stitches, I would not have peeked. I didn't want to look at it.

It was huge. Not wide and gaping, but longer than expected. Twice the length. Before surgery we were told it would run from your belly button to your groin. This scar started from the middle of your chest. It was clean, with staples running every half inch. It wasn't gross. Not at all. It was permanent. Permanence drawn in a pink-fleshy-stapled line as you fingered the wound.

"I just survived cancer."

EEE. EEE. EEE.

...

Farts, passing gas, BMs, and poopies—we detailed, deliberated, and celebrated each one as a glorious victory. Solid foods were consumed. Another victory. Pain medications lowered, tubes removed and bandages replaced. Your mother got you standing, walking, and sitting. We were told that exercise was very important to the recovery process. In only a week's time you could walk and eat and sit up. So many simple things to celebrate.

We made a routine out of the simple achievements. By Wednesday, I liked going for our nightly walk around the cancer ward. You shuffled in your slipper socks and hospital pajamas, leaning on your IV drip like a crutch. Do you remember the old lady with eyes the size of dinner plates from behind her coke-bottle glasses? She'd shoo us away as we passed, hollering, "You're making me look bad, son. Go back to bed." There was the father with prostate cancer who'd salute us every time we passed so he wouldn't interrupt his little boy reading aloud. And the old priest who came to visit the bearded fisherman with liver cancer; they'd both look up, in unison say, "God bless," pausing in mid-prayer.

I was proud of you. I never told you that then, but I was proud of that final crooked walk as we waved goodbye to the patients, plodding along toward recovery.

We hugged your mother goodbye at the airport, thankful our time at the hospital was over.

even if i am.

...

Tuesday, November 22
exit/enter

fuck.
so i walk out of the hospital,
or rather, i do a sad hunched/shuffle version
of the way i used to walk,
and i breathe the air like it's the first time,
and i smile at the sky like i'm seeing an old friend,
and its so cliché i have to laugh a little,
because i have become a hallmark card.

It's ten minutes since my victory lap around the fourth floor,
complete with high fives from the nurses
and goodbyes from the other patients,
thirty minutes since i was unplugged
from my last IV/attachment
and allowed to shower for the first time
since the morning of surgery,
six days since i entered this hospital
to live within its muted colors,
and it feels fucking great to finally be going home.

i walk to a nearby bench
to wait for chas to pull up the cruiser,
and sit with some effort,

EEE. EEE. EEE.

finding a posture that seems more akin
to a zen buddhist than a cancer patient, but it works
and it gives me a moment to think about it all.
cancer.
surgery.
friends.
family.
life.

all the words and all the advice echo
and i remember this is far from the end,
that in fact, there is no end.
i had cancer. they cut it out.
but even if it's not in me,
it will be a part of me.

other patients come in and out of the doors,
some sporting wheelchairs, others wearing obvious wigs.
this is my team?
can't we re-pick?

posted by Anthony Glass at 2:35 p.m.

chapter thirty

details of the war

I CREATED THIS ROMANTIC IDEA OF US, VERY AIR SUPPLY soft rock ballad, all agony and angsty. "Making Love Out of Nothing at All." I do that. When I meet someone, I create a story of what our life will be like together. It had a perfect beginning and a perfect end and it was beautiful. We were placed in treble clefs, sinking into the notes and simply letting go. There were no hospital beds or four-week recovery times, no swallowing pain medications or slathering ointments or guitar solos or drum machines. We were a love song, sweet as a melody. We were perfect instruments, strings flattering winds. We were perfect words, sung like poems. You had learned all the words to me, and I loved you like a favorite song.

Yet, I can't remember how the song goes without cancer. It seems a thousand years since the news. Anthony, you were still you, and I was still me, and our lives were still our lives, and it was still a love song. But one day I woke up, and I didn't recognize the tune. The beat wasn't the same. We certainly weren't the same song. I don't know why, we just were different. There were scarred guitar solos. Jaded refrains. Diseased tempos. I wanted to pick up the song where we left off, a sweet soft ballad of love.

For some piece of mind I threw myself into routine, envious you got to stay home and rest. Though, I hadn't made the connection that four-week's recovery meant you at home. I left, fully expecting to see you at work.

...

Monday, November 28
monday monday

woke up at 7 a.m., showered/shaved,
got dressed like i had somewhere to go,
and then sat myself down at the computer.
starting today, i work for myself.

made my to-do list:
contact the bank and hospital,
file for disability,
finish writing appeal to blue cross.

okay.
so working for yourself sucks.

planning on being out of work for four weeks, maybe more. three hours into it, and i'm already bored out of my skull. adding to my to-do list: "find a side project."

posted by Anthony Glass at 10:31 a.m.

...

I updated Kaethy, our boss, as vaguely as I could. "He's doing pretty good. I mean we've had a couple of health issues, but—yeah, he's doing well. He's having difficultly sleeping throughout the night, a lot of backaches but other than that... He just wants to be healing faster, so it can be over and done with." I wasn't going to tell her about your health setbacks, the bathroom accidents, or the lack of sleep. I cushioned the details, not just for her, but to everyone who asked. Even your parents. I knew they'd want to hear positives.

"But he's good. He's really good. You should read his blog. It gives you an update on how he's feeling."

"I tried to read it. I can't. It's too raw and too sad. I'm sorry. I'd rather hear it from you—sort of a buffer of news." Kaethy had become more of an older sister than a boss. You could feel it in her genuine concern and in her hugs. "I look forward to having him back at the office. I miss his smile. Everyone does."

"Yeah, me too."

even if i am.

. . .

From: le_samurai@yahoo.com
To: chasityrae@gmail.com
Sent: Tuesday, November 29, 4:30 p.m.
Subject: plans

just got back
from sending off my disability application to the dr.
went to the grocery store to buy some wet ones and soft TP,
ended up buying a bunch of everything...
getting ready to make some eggs and hash browns
for lunch...
yum.

miss you,
looking forward to cuddling tonight.

I didn't expect your body to go through cancer unchanged. I knew there would be physical scars, weight loss—all obvious changes I read about, but selfishly, I wanted you confident and aggressive. I wanted you sexy and always affectionate, the Anthony I knew you to be.

It was a challenge to stay physically connected. Not having sex didn't make it any easier. It made you feel insecure. You joked, "What thirty-year-old is too sick for sex?" I never once thought that cancer would affect my sex life. That seems absurdly self-serving, but it was a topic of concern. I was reluctant to bring it up. Hey, it's not like you brought it up, either, Anthony. I think we just both figured it would happen when it happened.

So, I stepped up my game. I needed to set the mood, set the stage. I lit a dozen candles. I cooked. Clearly I was up to something as I put on our favorite album, Ray Lamontange's *Trouble*. I wanted to renew our connection with some romantic music, something flawless, something hypnotic. The music had you on your feet, and you gracefully grabbed my hand and slowly twirled me into an embrace. I don't remember what song played. I can't remember if I was singing or humming or swaying along with your body against mine. I don't know if it was a sad song or one that made me want to turn up the volume as loud as it could go. There was music, though, and you were close enough to touch. That much I know.

"I miss feeling your body. I miss being close to you," I said in the middle of the chorus, my face burrowed in your chest.

"I miss being inside you." Your words tickled my neck. "Can you teach me again how you feel?"

I practically moaned.

You clutched my wrist, led me to the bedroom. Just breathe, I told myself. Breeeaaathe... I removed your clothes. Not fast. Not slow either. Then carefully slipped off my dress, letting it drop to the floor. Kissing the bare skin of your shoulder, you gently pushed me back onto the bed. I was speechless, arching to feel your body. I hesitated. I wondered if it was unhealthy if my body touched yours, your incision. I didn't want to cause pain or discomfort or infection. I didn't want to squish you or hurt you or rub too rough. You too hesitated, unsure of what move to make next, cautious of your bare skin touching my belly, your exposed scar laid carefully on top of me. Neither of us moved, afraid it might be injurious.

"If my senses fail, don't be mad at me," you whispered tenderly. "I just want to feel you again."

My heart was temporarily suspended in the sentence as your fingers trailed from my brow around my cheek to my chin. We were completely connected, completely free.

"You feel perfect. Exactly as I remember." My voice barely a whisper.

...

From: le_samurai@yahoo.com
To: chasityrae@gmail.com
Sent: Wednesday, November 30, 7:00 p.m.
Subject: feeling better

showered and dressed at your place,
decided to come home
and mail the doctor's checks from home (don't ask)
and i ate a couple bowls of cereal when i got here,
wrote the checks out and immediately felt like shit.
staggered to the post office
to send the envelopes out,

and then came home and passed out
for about four hours...

got up a little while ago,
feeling better,
still gross, but better,
and i'm getting my appetite back...
but what should i eat?

and that part of me that i was complaining about this morning
is still driving me fucking nuts!
It's my upper left leg...
tingly pain... fuck!

sorry it took me so long to write,
but i hope you're having a good day,
and not worrying about me too much...

it was a nice morning of cuddling,
and a good way to start a day
that just couldn't quite keep up...

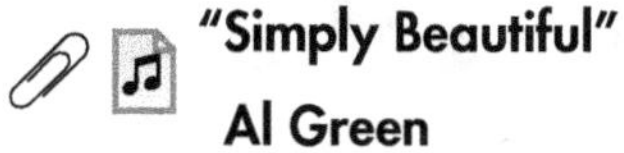

...

There's no use in wondering why a bad day leads to a fight. You were discouraged and you didn't want me to see that you were not improving anymore. You turned away, took the bad nights alone. You'd blow up over petty things, like whether I changed the toilet paper roll and how. I know your anger didn't mean you no longer loved me. People are terrible to the ones they love sometimes. They're mean for no reason at all. And for my part, I was mean. I yelled back.

"Change the goddamn roll yourself!"

I instantly regretted yelling, but it was already out of my mouth. Ours was not the worst relationship in the world. Other couples fight about stupid things, right? It's just that we were all we had. We depended on each other, every moment of every day and we expected a lot. Worse, it was difficult to enjoy the moments in between the bickering and simply forget ourselves.

I kept trying to pick up the pieces, waiting for a hint of a spark of something outside of cancer.

"C'mon let's go for a walk," I said, pulling you off the couch.

"I am so fucking tired. I just want to go to bed."

Regretting it before I even said it, "You know, I need you to rally for me, too. Not just for your family on the phone or your friends, but for me, too! Just give me something good, one goddamn good night, that isn't about cancer and feeling like shit and being tired or crabby or any other excuse you can think of."

You tuned out and said nothing.

...

Thursday, December 1
so, yesterday sucked.

ate two bowls of cereal in the morning,
and it completely knocked me into nasty.
felt all bad things while trying to function,
and finally surrendered to a four-hour nap.
(is four hours still considered a nap?)
i watched a movie, and spent the rest of the day
in a grouchy, vegetative state.
yeeeesh.
needless to say,
i'm planning out my diet today
with a little more discretion.

i know there will be more bad days,
that they're part of the process:
expecting anything else is naive.
but in recovery you get used to progress,
accustomed to improvement,
so much so that when you take a step back
it feels like it's so much farther than it is.

even if i am.

this morning,
showered.
rested.
a long list of things to do,
things that will get done
instead of slept on.
people to call back.
out of minutes on my phone, but fuck it…

make today as good
as yesterday was bad.

It's all part of the process.

posted by Anthony Glass at 8:17 a.m.

From: le_samurai@yahoo.com
To: chasityrae@gmail.com
Sent: Thursday, December 1, 12:05 p.m.
Subject: this morning

made my list of things,
showered.
clean.

wrote a new entry in my blog,
planning on writing more later for myself.

nothing inspires a good day
more than a bad one.

it seems you have the bad shift again...
coming to see me at night,
after the day has taken its toll on me,
and i have nothing left to offer
except sad, confused stories from the day
and an exhausted head in your lap.
that sucks.

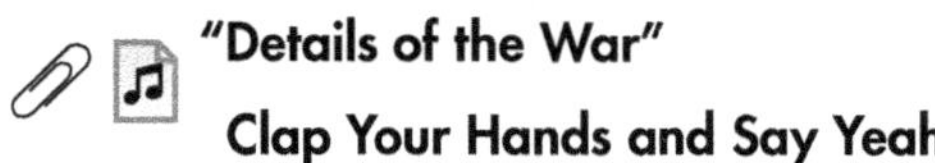
"Details of the War"
Clap Your Hands and Say Yeah

"I just want to see you happy again," I told your voicemail. "We all just want to see you happy again—your family, your friends, your girlfriend, Gladys... That's all I was trying to do. I'll call you later tonight when I get home. I miss you."

chapter thirty-one

song for a sleeping girl

You spent a great deal of time drafting an appeal letter to Blue Cross. I didn't understand why it was so time consuming. It wasn't until you asked your parents and me to proofread it that I understood the burden.

From: le_samurai@yahoo.com
To: mother
stepfather
chasityrae@gmail.com
Sent: Friday, December 2, 3:03 p.m.
Subject: appeal letter

Dear Blue Cross Person:

My name is Anthony Glass. I am 30 years old, and in August I was diagnosed with advanced stage 3 rectal cancer.

It was finally the answer to questions I had been asking, complaints I had been giving to a variety of physicians, for over five years. My symptoms had been disregarded by my doctors, and consequently, disregarded by me. It was a hard lesson to learn, but one that taught me that my health is my responsibility. When I was referred to a general surgeon to perform my coloanal anastamosis, a surgeon who was not board-certified in colorectal surgery, I felt it was my responsibility to find a specialist.

Dr. Beart, the chief of colo-rectal surgery at the USC Norris Cancer Hospital is one of the leading specialists in the country. He is a board-certified colorectal surgeon, and treats cases like mine on a regular basis. However, my referral to him was denied by my medical group.

Unfortunately, this was no surprise. When I was first diagnosed, I asked to be referred to a nutritionist so that I could modify my diet to suit my condition, and help prepare me for the rigors of chemo/radiation therapy, as well as surgery. The referral was denied. Although I don't understand the logic behind denying a cancer patient a meeting with a nutritionist, I accepted the decision. However, a surgeon is another matter.

I am writing to appeal the decision to deny Dr. Beart as my surgeon, and ask for Blue Cross to assume the responsibility it owes to me in providing me with the kind of care my health requires.

Thank you for your consideration,
Anthony Glass

— Forwarded Message to chasityrae@gmail.com
From: stepfather
To: mother
le_samurai@yahoo.com
chasityrae@gmail.com
Sent: Saturday, December 3, 5:21 a.m.
Subject: Re: appeal letter

Hi, Anth. I have a few editorial comments on your Blue Cross appeal, below. It was easier to rewrite it than to change your version, which was a good take-off point. It will seem to the medical director that you may have had help in writing this. That is not a bad thing, as he will see that you are backed up and well advised, and he may even worry a little about adverse publicity or malpractice action. He is well enough paid that a little worry is part of his job description.

I hope your recovery continues, and each day is better than the last. It is encouraging that you are eating real food and doing a little work from home. Whatever is going well can of course be attributed to the excellent nursing care given to you by Chas.

We think of you often and you are always in our prayers.

Love,
Dad

To: Medical Director
Subject: Appeal of disallowed out-of-plan services

I, Anthony Glass (age 30) have been diagnosed with Colorectal adenocarcinoma, stage 3.

I believe that I have not been well served by my health plan and have been forced into getting out-of-plan care for which I have personally paid $36,550, which I can ill afford. My previous request for coverage was denied, and I could not wait, in the face of advancing cancer, for prolonged wrangling with Blue Cross.

Failure to diagnose: I have had bowel dysfunction for over five years and have made repeated visits to my plan physicians, only to be reassured that it was nothing to worry about: this, despite diarrhea and blood in the stools for many months. Finally, at my insistence, a colonoscopy revealed cancer and imaging studies showed multiple lymph node involvement. A program of local irradiation with chemotherapy adjunct, then surgery, and then chemotherapy, was recommended and commenced.

Disallowed services: I had significant problems with diarrhea and was facing radiation, surgery, and chemotherapy. Therefore I requested consultation with a nutritionist to avoid making my condition worse by wrong food selection and to build myself up for this ordeal. It was disallowed.

More significant, I was referred to a general surgeon for this major colorectal cancer surgery. In getting a second opinion, I became aware that colorectal cancer surgery is a boarded surgical subspecialty, and that USC has a center designed for this purpose which handles a large number of such cases. I requested authorization to have my surgery there and it was disallowed.

The surgery has been performed, and involved dissection about the rectum at the pelvic brim, removal of a segment of colon and regional lymph nodes, primary re-anastomosis, and extensive dissection in removing a large, tumor-containing node which lay just under the left kidney and rested on the aorta and renal vein. My surgeon was Dr. Beart, chief of colorectal surgery at the USC Norris Cancer Hospital. I feel I had the benefit of state-of-the-art surgical care. However, I was required to personally pay $36,550 up front, out of pocket, to avoid having my surgery cancelled. It seems that Blue Cross was toying with my life and my future by only allowing a general surgeon in a non-cancer center for this specialized procedure.

Request: Accordingly, I request that my out-of-pocket expenses for the surgery be allowed and reimbursed by my Blue Cross plan, and that I be covered for surgical follow-up with Dr. Beart and his group.

Thank you for your sympathetic consideration.
Anthony Glass

"I read your stepfather's letter. It's concise, I'll give it that."

"Yeah. It's rather formal sounding, but if he thinks it's what we should send to my health insurance…" Your voice was hoarse over the phone. "Oh, I got a call from the hospital, checking in. I couldn't think of anything bad to report, so I told the doctor I was doing fine."

"Did you mention your tingling leg?" This was the only symptom I could think of, even though there were a dozen more.

"No, it hasn't been bothering me."

"Well, that's good…" My tone deflated.

"Sooo?"

"Yeah?"

"I bought a Baja guidebook at the promenade today and am geeking out thinking about all the different ways we can spend Christmas together? What do think? Christmas in

Mexico?" I could feel your excitement through the phone. You were eager to share a spark of something good.

"I thought you'd never ask." I said through a smile.

"I'm waiting for Zach to call me back, I get the feeling he wants to hang out tonight. Maybe you should come over anyway, and I can show you the book while we all watch the football game? Yes? Maybe? One big happy family? Football and Baja?"

"As long as you cuddle with me and not Zach."

...

Monday, December 5
this is what it's like to be at home sick

1. the days go by infinitely faster.
   it's frickin' monday again? really?

2. puritanical work ethic = guilt
   whenever someone calls, i feel compelled to give them detailed accounts of what i've done with my time, and the things i have accomplished, even if its utterly asinine "...and then i changed from my walking shoes, to my house shoes... mmm, comfy they are!"

3. what have i done?
   secretly, i thought this recovery period could be recalled in later years by scholars as "anthony's most prolific

creative period, a time from which his genius was truly unleashed..." rather than a time in which he watched movies and took walks and short naps.

4. man becomes dog.
   i feel myself coming to understand the relationship dogs have with the mailman: when you're least expecting it, all of a sudden, there's someone AT YOUR DOOR! i can see his shadow, the lid on my mailbox slams, and then he's gone! such an invasion of privacy, i almost barked this morning. just take my netflix and go!

5. i have become one of them.
   there was always a mystery to the masses of people i would see mulling about when everyone else was working (and no, i'm not just talking about the homeless). i mean the cult of people who hang out at the coffee bean on an idle tuesday afternoon, the small mass of hipsters shuffling along abbott kinney boulevard, seeming to have no destination or time frame. they can't all be actors, can they? walking on the promenade early this afternoon, i looked into a storefront window, and in the reflection (gasp!) saw that i had become one of them.

do you think they all have cancer too?

posted by Anthony Glass at 6:18 p.m.

...

I was half awake for a good chunk of the night, enduring that in-between state of confusion and wakefulness and fatigue. So, I just lay in bed trying to sleep, thinking of us in Mexico. I played it out like a daydream, making it up as it went along: lying on a deserted beach, salt water shedding our winter skin.

You slept fitfully next to me. Seriously, you're the worst sleeper. EVER. I imagined you sleeping soundly and quietly next to me on a beach in Mexico, fully surrendering to the lullaby of the receding tide. Then, the dream took a turn, to us on a rocky boat at sea, drowning as waves crashed over me.

It was just your arm twitching on top of my shoulders.

"Babe, try to get some sleep."

...

From: le_samurai@yahoo.com
To: chasityrae@gmail.com
Sent: Tuesday, December 6, 6:21 p.m.
Subject: the kind of thing

just got back from riding down to the beach,
ate some lunch and sat on the grass looking out at the ocean.
the kind of thing one thinks one would do
if one had a day off from work.

even if i am.

it doesn't sound like a lot,
but i ate the whole sandwich and bag of chips.
felt a little like i'm getting my appetite back.

made some basic grammatical changes to the letter,
and filled in some missing info, but other than that,
i just don't feel connected to it.
read my old letter, and started to feel like
perhaps i'm sending the wrong letter.
i guess if everyone prefers my stepfather's letter,
then it's the one i should be sending to Blue Cross,
but i just don't feel like it's my words.

despite it all, i am feeling much better.

i miss you.

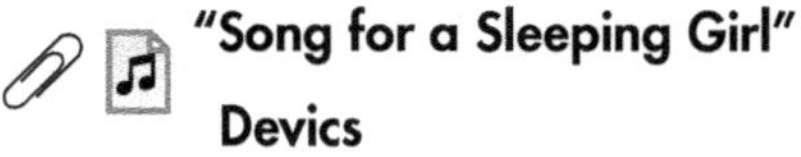

...

I'm not even sure I was a good caregiver—not that you didn't compliment me, but I struggled to keep up with everyday life. It was hard work, caregiving. Overwhelming work. Yet, I was determined I could handle this myself; full-time job, bills, laundry, grocery shopping, dishes, yard work, not to mention keeping up with Gladys. Anyway, it was temporary. Things would get back to the way they were. They'd be even better.

Everyone wanted to know how I was doing, as if it were the only question that mattered. When I ran into Zach at the office, whom I hadn't seen hardly at all, he asked, "How are you?" I smiled like a politician and stated, "I am good. Things are very good." It was the only answer I ever gave, because I knew it was the one people wanted to hear.

"Hey, you guys wanna go to an art show tomorrow night? It's on Abbott Kinney. I'll come pick you up…"

…

From: le_samurai@yahoo.com
To: chasityrae@gmail.com
Sent: Thursday, December 8, 1:02 p.m.
Subject: rough night

rough night last night,
took a couple of aleves, and then rolled around
quite a bit before finally falling asleep.
woke up a couple of times,
but just couldn't get comfy.

glad to hear we're going to the art opening tonight.
i think it'll be fun for us to do something like that
(jeez, i hope the art is cool.)

even if i am.

i'll see if jay wants to come, and make it a foursome.

i promise i'll come out to your side of town this weekend.
you've been making the commute quite a bit.

one thing i do miss about being at work
is knowing that at any given moment
you could be at my door, in my office,
and we could be sharing a big and beautiful embrace.

miss you lots.

It was as if someone told Zach, "Don't mention the cancer. It's too depressing. Just try to be upbeat." He talked football. With him we didn't talk disease or recovery time; we talked Redskins and basketball and movies and art. He meant well, but it gave the conversation an unreal cast. Cancer didn't define who you were by any means, but it was filling up your days. From the books you read, to the discussions you had, to advice that you were given, even to reasons people were getting in touch with you, it defined your everyday routines. Cancer became a part of your identity, but it didn't define who you were.

song for a sleeping girl

...

Friday, December 9
slaying my dragons

the back door is open, the sun shining in
(is that a warm breeze i detect?)
put the headphones on,
time to write.

listening to my new favorite band: clap your hands say yeah!
quite sure they are now forever linked to this period of my life.

things are improving. daily.
went to an art opening last night with some friends,
and even managed to go to a nearby bar afterwards
to share some wine, and talk snot about art and life.

however, i do think i'm getting an early taste
of what it will be like when i'm old:
after standing and walking for a while, i was pooped.
i had to search out a place to sit and rest:
"no you guys go ahead, i just need to sit down for a
moment..."

putting away the puzzle that chas and i assembled
(okay it really was all her...
she is FREAKISH with those things!)

even if i am.

decided to take a quick pic of it
before returning to its original state
(it glows in the dark,
but the camera couldn't quite get an exposure).
if you can't quite tell from the picture,
its a knight on a flying unicorn,
slaying a medallion-wearing dragon in an underwater cave.
fucking awesome.
thanks to charlie for a great get-well present.

yes, things are getting better:
one piece at a time.

...

From: le_samurai@yahoo.com
To: chasityrae@gmail.com
Sent: Friday, December 9, 12:11 p.m.
Subject: art

are you cursing my name this morning.
sleepwalking to work,
wondering aloud why you allowed yourself
to stay out late on the westside once again?

hope not.

i slept better than usual,

although i woke up at some mysterious hour,
and stumbled into the kitchen for some water
only to find jay passed out at the computer
head resting on keyboard.

it was a little sad, but i didn't have the heart to wake him.
needless to say, i can't wait to see if he has "asdfghjkl"
tattooed to his forehead this morning.
i had fun last night.
looking at art with you and zach,
and then finding our cozy corner to sit at the bar.
that was a nice evening.

Jay should have been our third wheel. After all, he's your best friend and roommate. Yet I haven't even included him in this story. Truth is, Jay wasn't around much. His emotions were ensnared in heartbreak and girls, and the fallout from his latest breakup had manifested in a pattern of isolation and drinking. Roommate trouble seems part and parcel with being in your twenties—but was it a good excuse? It was hard to not take it personally, wondering why your best friend was missing during your healing. From an outsider's perspective, I understood his distance. Hell, I envied it. While you were his rock, I honestly don't think he knew how to be yours.

"So, Jay and I finally talked last night. We put a lot of things out on the table, but focused mostly on how he's been completely absent from my recovery and wrapped up in his own shit. It was frustrating, emotional, and ultimately a conversation we should have had a while ago. It ended with him in tears, apologizing, and both of us feeling a sense of relief—but he's also having a lot of things to deal with."

"Like what?"

"He is afraid of life and death, depressed his best friend has cancer. He doesn't know how to deal with these things. He doesn't know how to be a friend. He said so. That it's a heartbreaking situation and scary situation and he doesn't know how to deal with that kind of stuff. He's not good at that kind of stuff..."

chapter thirty-two

a change at christmas

From: le_samurai@yahoo.com
To: chasityrae@gmail.com
Sent: Tuesday, December 13, 3:55 p.m.
Subject: early

arrived a little early to the doctor's office,
sat around for a bit until they called me.
(it was a little nostalgic to be back.)

walked to one of the exam rooms
with the doctor and assistant.
on the way, we stopped at a scale and weighed in
(this time only wearing a tee shirt and jeans, no shoes),
came in around 178 pounds.

don't think i've weighed that little since high school,
maybe junior high.

even if i am.

the assistant gave me a gown
and asked me to change (oh great)
and then i sat in the exam room and waited for a doctor
for at least thirty minutes. (in a frickin gown!)

doctor came in, asked me a couple of questions,
then another doctor came in flustered
like she was running late,
and they ended up both discussing the surgery with me
took a look at the incision, complimented me on it,
referred me to the oncologist to talk about the chemo,
asked to see me again in four months (why, i don't know)
and that was it.
no anal probe!
but an utterly purposeless visit.

came home and watched "the burbs" with jay,
passed out for a spell in my bed.
don't know why i'm so tired.

getting ready to run out and grab some lunch.
am i going to waste this day as well?
hope not. hope some food will give me energy.

and you?
how are you holding up today?
missing me?

be well,
write when you can.

From: chasityrae@gmail.com
To: le_samurai@yahoo.com
Sent: Tuesday, December 13, 6:26 p.m.
Subject: Re: early

sounds like another fun visit to the doctor's.
they complimented you on your scar?
that's fantastic.
178 POUNDS! You NEED to eat more throughout the day!

I'm worried about you...
and I sorta feel like Ms. Claus yelling at Santa:
"Eat, Papa. Eat! No one likes a skinny Santa."

...

I worked late, then drove to your house. I sneaked through the back door, slipped under the blankets and behind you. My plan was to lay awake and listen to you breathing, listen to the night before everything woke up. You were my little spoon in the darkness, as I buried the front off my knees into the back of yours, my tummy nestled against your arch, my nose in the curve of your neck, I kissed your hair. "I am happy," I mumbled softy.

"What are you doing here?" you said, somehow pulling me closer.

"I know it's late, but I couldn't imagine another night without you next to me. I'm happy."

"I think you should move in."

"You're half asleep."

"Move in with me."

"Will you wake up in the morning and remember what you just asked me?"

"Probably not, but move in with me anyway, I feel better when you're here."

...

From: le_samurai@yahoo.com
To: chasityrae@gmail.com
Sent: Wednesday, December 14, 12:49 p.m.
Subject: fuzzy

i have this fuzzy memory of you last night,
perhaps it was a dream,
but you showed up out of nowhere
and rolled around in bed with me for a while.

after you left i actually slept very well
(didn't get up once although i would have
gotten up for water if it wasn't so cold out).
jay just left for work, which usually means

that i'll get a lot of stuff done.

are you sleepy?
must've gotten home very late.
thank you for the surprise, it was delightful.

From: chasityrae@gmail.com
To: le_samurai@yahoo.com
Sent: Wednesday, December 14, 1:17 a.m.
Subject: Re: fuzzy

last night was fun.
I like surprise visits.
I like throwing you off,
crawling into bed,
spilling secrets and cuddling.

do you remember what you asked me?

From: le_samurai@yahoo.com
To: chasityrae@gmail.com
Sent: Wednesday, December 14, 5:19 p.m.
Subject: Re: fuzzy

finished everything for my HMO appeal,
drove out to kinkos, made the copies i needed,
paperclipped everything so it was perfectly organized,
and as i was sliding it into an envelope,

even if i am.

i noticed a giant typo in my opening letter.
fuck.

so i'm back home now,
reprinting and running back out.
but realized i hadn't sent you an afternoon e-mail
(or a song yet for that matter, a christmas song).

i think christmas shopping is the first way
to start getting into the spirit of the season,
but my favorite one is to find a list of the best
decorated christmas light houses in LA
and then drive around and look at them.
we should do that when our social calendar clears...
january maybe?

putting my christmas list together,
and getting excited about it.
i feel a little lucky to be home,
and presumably to have time off
to get some of this stuff done.
but time's running out!

okay, i'm off to kinko's again,
can't wait to be all done with blue cross
(again, for the time being).

fucking love the shit out of you.

yes, i remember what i asked.

"A Change At Christmas (Say It Isn't So)"
Death Cab for Cutie

You rarely mentioned the low periods or health concerns to your mother or stepfather or friends. I got the brunt of it. "Yeah, last night was a hard one. I couldn't sleep at all. My back was killing me. I didn't know you stayed up so late—that makes it even crappier."

"It's okay." I tried not to sound as exhausted as the sentence felt. "Just tired."

"I kept waking up, hot, uncomfortable. It was better after Gladys went into the living room but I felt sad, like you were cut off for some reason. I hate when we have nights like that. I like it better when we wake up, cuddle, and fall back asleep."

"Me, too. Sorry if I felt cut off. I just thought you were sleeping well, and I didn't want to keep waking you—your back hurt again? That sucks. I know you're having a hard time sleeping as it is. I should have cuddled anyway." I wished I answered in a pithier manner. "I miss your cuddles."

"It'll be interesting to see how we sleep together in a strange bed over the holidays…"

"OHHH! I can't wait for Mexico!" I squealed, and turned on my charm. "Who says we're sleeping?"

even if i am.

...

From: le_samurai@yahoo.com
To: chasityrae@gmail.com
Sent: Monday, December 19, 3:12 p.m.
Subject: mexico

hot fucking shit!
we have a reservation in room 18,
one that the travelogue recommended,
which has an ocean view and a fireplace.
checking in between 3 p.m. and 5 p.m. on the 23rd,
and then checking out before noon on the 26th.

you can also do a search for "hotel la fonda baja"
and see all the travelogue sites that come up.
we're fucking celebrating, right?

i miss you, too.
getting tons done,
like wrapping presents.

From: chasityrae@gmail.com
To: le_samurai@yahoo.com
Sent: Monday, December 19, 11:26 p.m.
Subject: Re: mexico

I want you to know

a change at christmas

that I think about you
every chance I get.
that I catch myself wondering what you are up to.
I catch myself smiling
even laughing out loud
thinking of you.

I daydream of our trip to Mexico
while trying to focus on work...

and I wanted you to know,
that no matter how busy my day is,
no matter how sleepy I am,
or how few e-mails I respond to...

I wanted you to know,
I love you.

and I wish I could show you
just how much I loved you
every second of every day.

...

It wasn't the gorgeous drive over the border, or the songs we sung while driving the coast. It wasn't the perfect hotel view or the couples' massage. It was Christmas morning.

Christmas Eve had swallowed us like the horizon swallowed the sun, plunging us into a long, languid night. We tried to stay quiet when hotel guests slept in the next room; felt the agony of trying not to laugh when our bed slid or we both wanted to scream. I remember our half-asleep talk of living together as we rolled around in todays and tomorrows. And then—Christmas morning, I remember waking to the trace of tiny kisses sneaking their way from my mouth to my tummy. You were in my bloodstream, crawling in and out of my heart, my veins, making it difficult for me to get the words out and simply wish you a Merry Christmas. I closed my eyes again, hoping my anticipation wouldn't wake you. I thought about cancer and us and moving in together after the holidays and surgery and Mexico and the universe and all of the things I was grateful for.

Was it really only yesterday we drew our names in the sand and warmed our feet by the fire and shared words of hope? I wanted to do it all again, but you looked so sweet as the bar of morning light warmed your shoulder, strands of my hair still wrapped around your finger. I couldn't wait a second longer.

"Good morning you. Merry Christmas," I sang.

"You're still here?" you muttered under my thousand and one kisses to your dry lips.

"Where else would I be?"

"Opening presents."

Waking in white sheets with our legs wrapped around each other, my face resting on your chest, we seemed to fully become the time and place. Wrapped only in sheets and blankets, we handed out presents. You gave me the sweetest gift ever. (No. Not that one.) I can't believe you had saved every e-mail I ever sent you, from the very first till the very last. It must have taken you weeks to compile such a present. It was perfect, the most beautiful collection of all the e-mails we sent, cut and pasted into a used art book of pencil sketches by an unknown artist. You titled it simply, "Us."

chapter thirty-three

in the sun

Saturday, January 7
in the middle

halftime?
intermission?
c'mon glass, there's an analogy here somewhere...

with some argument from my insides, i can say now
that i have completely recovered from the surgery.
i am walking, moving, and living just like i used to.
and it's fucking great.

most times, the thoughts of cancer, of surgery, of everything,
recedes to the back of my head,
and quietly lies down for a nap.
but they wake easily.
running my hand across my belly,

even if i am.

there's a twelve inch reminder:
of the weeks past, of the months ahead.

visited the oncologist this week and got my chemo recipe:
one two-hour IV treatment of oxyplatinum every three weeks,
two pills of xoloda taken twice a day between treatments,
six cycles.
simmer.
for best results add supplements during treatment.

so here we are,
and i still don't have a metaphor.
the short break before the last climb?
ewey, that's cheeseball.
the deep breath before… aw gad, that's worse.

honestly, it sucks to start over again.
to have worked back to feeling normal,
and to have to give that up.
but the last couple of weeks have been great,
and if anything, they are a reminder of what
it will be like after these six cycles are done.
that is something to look forward to.
on that note, i've included a picture from christmas in mexico:
chas and i warming our feet by the fireplace.
yum.

posted by Anthony Glass at 7:43 a.m.

...

I'm a pretty girl. I'm not trying to sound vain. Though, I think that is all your mother sees in me—the blonde hair, the pretty face. I'm not smart or talented or even interesting. I didn't graduate from college. I can't believe I told her that. "I was getting far more experience working than through education." I wish hadn't said that. She went through grad school supporting three growing boys, and I made it seem as if an education wasn't important. Ugh. I'm just another pretty girl among all the girls she's met before.

I don't want you to think I hated her. I don't hate her. It's just when she came to visit for a random weekend, she tried to make up for the weeks she hadn't been here. She'd fly into town for a biopsy or scan, stay for two days, then fly home. Babe, I'm sorry, but her visits were tiresome. She'd tell me what we needed to do for your health, what vitamins you should take, what your calorie count should be. Do you remember when she taught me how to properly rub your back, on your back? She moved my hand from your shoulder in order to show me the pressure points. "Apply pressure to both sides of the spine like this. Use your fingers and move your way upward to his skull." My palm turned clammy with embarrassment. I didn't know anything about pressure points. I started doubting myself. I didn't even know how to rub your back right. What if loving you wasn't enough? She could do that. In two days, she could somehow make me feel like a crappy girlfriend. I needed to do more, cook healthier, rub your back harder.

Okay, maybe I was starting to hate her. Why wasn't she here more? Her son had cancer, for God's sake! I was attending every follow-up, every treatment, every holistic opinion, doing everything I could possibly do. So what if I didn't know how to cook broccoli in the stupid microwave?

...

From: le_samurai@yahoo.com
To: chasityrae@gmail.com
Sent: Tuesday, January 10, 5:45 p.m.
Subject: hello there

i'm getting into the shower,
and my mom is sitting at the puzzle.
i wish you were here to help her with the puzzle,
and tickle me as i get into the shower.

so, my mom and i have been discussing the merits
of switching to the PPO versus staying with my HMO,
and i think i'm going to stick with the HMO
(assuming i am still able to do so).

with all the chemo i will be taking for the next few months
and potential follow-ups in the months following,
it seems like it makes sense financially to stay HMO.

you can imagine how much fun we're having discussing it.
up next: 401k.
i need you here.
now.
help.
buffer.
something…

hope your day is going well.
you really should get here soon,
i might kill her before long…

i fuckin' love the fuck out of you.

work hard.
see you soon.

From: chasityrae@gmail.com
To: le_samurai@yahoo.com
Sent: Tuesday, January 10, 6:15 p.m.
Subject: mom

have a good day with your mom today.
she is trying to help…
but yes, it will be wonderful to drive her to the airport tonight.
(did I just type that?)

know that I am thinking of you. like always.
(mmm, to tickle you...)

...

You returned to work, and we picked up our old routine where we left off. We forgave quickly, kissed slowly, laughed uncontrollably. I thanked God on drives home. Held heavenly conversations of gratitude. It was hard to believe only eleven months of strange steps traced back to the beginning.

Babe, we are a story about love, not cancer. Our chapters ended sweetly with the four simple words, I fucking love you. We believed that there was so much ahead of us that we had no need to look back at old chapters. We talked about cancer less. Our lips were fat with kisses and the words I love you. We let our smiles twist and turn, just wanting to be together. When chemo started I barely noticed the change in each day.

From: le_samurai@yahoo.com
To: chasityrae@gmail.com
Sent: Monday, January 16, 7:30 p.m.
Subject: hmmmm...

how this day has gotten away from us.
no e-mail?
maybe because i've been obsessed with
going through my footage

and finishing this edit;
or maybe it's because you came in this morning,
looking so fresh and so beautiful,
you kind of knocked me out a bit.

finally got some good news
from the last project.
the client loved it
and kaethy even read the e-mail out loud
to give me the good news verbatim.
nice.

now if i can just do something brilliant
with this new project.
how was the rest of your day?
why haven't you come by to give me
any more kisses/loving/sweetness?

p.s. kisses and touching in the stairwell was nice. i like being back at work.

...

I never liked needles or hospitals, and especially not needles at hospitals. I don't even like watching Gladys get a shot from the vet; the technician grabs her leash, and I stay in the waiting room, feeling like a bad mother. With you, I did not have the luxury of being squeamish. The quality of love and reciprocity changed everything. I could watch them connect and disconnect the intravenous chemo. I could watch the needles pierce your skin, no problem. I saw it. I didn't turn. I didn't faint. I could even pull the sticky bandages off your hairy arm. My mom once told me that "God doesn't give you anything you can't handle." I don't know what God has to do with this, but it made me feel better when I pulled off your Band Aids and kissed your hurts.

...

You nicknamed him Dr. Apathy. His smile was detached. His hair was nonchalant, even his clothes were drab. I will grant that administering chemo to patients five days a week is not a job in which to invest much emotion, but every visit made us feel like a paycheck, not a patient. He even rescheduled one of your treatments to attend his daughter's soccer game. His patients were fighting for their lives, and he was more concerned about missing a soccer game? Crook.

His waiting room was so full that he set up your chemo in his office and plopped you on his couch. Babe, I still don't know how you could sit in the waiting room and thumb through the books filling the shelves, *American Cancer Society: Guide to Cancer Drugs, Second Edition*; *Everyone's Guide to Cancer Therapy*; *The Cancer Book*; *Informed Decisions.* I merely stared at the pictures of Dr. Apathy with his family vacationing, celebrating holidays, marking key moments of a healthy family. Enough photos to witness two beautiful daughters mature from babies, to high school, to college. The pictures annoyed me. Can you believe he had the nerve to answer his phone and make dinner plans with his wife? In front of us?

Whether we liked him or not, we didn't have a choice. He was your HMO. I couldn't help but laugh at the ridiculousness of the whole damn thing.

...

"Let's run away for your birthday," I said. I wanted to be snuggling and asking you in person, not over the phone.

"No, that's okay. I was thinking of just going to dinner, inviting some friends. Plus, we have chemo on Tuesday."

"It's not a question," I said. "The boat leaves at ten a.m. and it's a hour-long ride. We both have Monday off, so it'll be a three-day weekend. I already packed snacks and your suitcase..."

"Really, go away for my birthday? Where are we going?"

"Catalina is the farthest I could get us out of the country..."

Your laugh was loud. "I fucking love you."

"I love you more. Happy Birthday, baby."

even if i am.

...

Tuesday, January 24
it is a happy birfday

sitting down to write.
it's cold.
i'm tired.

not ideal conditions.

my memory walks to the fridge and opens a beer.
a place writers have found inspiration since writing began.
but these are not those times.
so instead, i walk to the stove and boil water.
pour a cup of green tea.
and sit down again.

it was my birthday yesterday.
31 years old.
i'm comfortable with my age.
confident with my life.
but let's be honest, not a sexy number.
it's odd, unbalanced, sharing none of the glory
that it's younger brother "21" wields.
no, not sexy at all.

my last few birthdays have been celebrated

by traveling someplace new, and (usually) someplace far.
however, as i've burned through all my vacation/sick days
for what may be the next five years, this year would be
different.

chas and i continued my fledgling tradition
by taking a ferry from long beach harbor
to catalina island (all of one whole hour away).
officially, we stepped off the mainland and therefore
traveled "overseas" to what honestly feels like a faraway land.
golf carts are the dominant mode of transportation.
buffalo roam in force.
old people are everywhere.
(a great place for feeling young.)

biggest changes i've made now that i'm 31:

1. new e-mail address. (a whole different story.)
2. use cnn.com for my news/info gathering. why?
   york did it, so it must be mature.
3. and beer is now tea. (see above.)

other than that, things are still very much the same.
and it is a happy birthday.

posted by Anthony Glass at 9:08 p.m.

even if i am.

From: anthonyglass@gmail.com
To: friends
Sent: Monday, January 25, 9:25 p.m.
Subject: true story

1996.
an impressionable young film student
saunters across the campus of san diego state,
and into the campus computer lab
to start an "e-mail account."

user ID? hmmm...
i could use my name?
no way, too unoriginal.
i'm a FILM student! be creative!

well, i just saw this great french film: le samorai.
it's different...
mysterious...
whatever.
i'll come up with something better tomorrow.

ten years later.
my girlfriend and i watch the recently issued dvd release
of the 1967 jean-pierre melville french gangster classic.
she falls asleep in the first act.
the plot twist makes no sense.
credits roll.

i am confused.
it dawns on me that for ten years i have carried the moniker of a film that i don't really understand,
and only marginally enjoy.
my girlfriend laughs.

i've been planning on starting a gmail account for some time, and well, frankly, this seems like the perfect time.
user ID?
anthonyglass@gmail.com.
write me anytime.

p.s. i have the dvd if anyone wants to borrow it and explain the end to me.

...

"Do you feel that?" you asked.

I placed my fingers under yours to examine your neck. "Where?"

"Right here," guiding my fingertips to the exact spot.

"Move your fingers. Right there?"

"Yeah?" I could feel the lump.

"It's hard. Like a little pea. What is it?"

"It's probably a swollen lymph node," I said in my best nurse voice. "Do you feel okay?"

"I feel a little tired, but not sick or anything."

even if i am.

“Do you think it’s a side effect from your chemo? Is it sore?”

“Not really. We should tell Dr. Apathy on Tuesday.”

“It’s probably nothing, but yeah let’s definitely tell him.”

…

Sunday, February 5
sparks

fuckin’ hell.
i should be writing more often than this.
it’s a fight.
but sundays are a day of surrender.
and sunday night, even more so.

this week was an ordinary week.
a good week.
full of work, chas, friends, stuff,
exercise. fuckin’ shit. raquetball?
it is quite a moment at 30 years old
(oh shit, 31 years old),
to admit to yourself you’ve never been
as out of shape in your life as you are now.
fuckin’ hell.

stretch.
remember.

in the sun

body.
strength.

okay, so it's superbowl sunday.
10 p.m.
the smoky aftermath is blowing by.
jay and i sold our souls to costco, home depot, and albertson's
so that we could pull a barbecue out of our arse...
and it was fucking worth it.
completely.
steaks. ahi. skewers. beer n' guacamole. what was forgotten?

it was a great group of people to balance the game,
the food, and the mutherfucking commercials...
commercials.
when does one pee?
miss the game or miss the culture?

guilty confession #1:
completely sold on the promos during the game,
ended up watching "grey's anatomy" after the game.
tried to find the michael stipe and coldplay cover
of "in the sun"
they used in the episode—too bad. too new.
listened to joseph arthur as we cleaned up the house.
listening to coldplay now.
feels like talking to an old friend.

even if i am.

strange how that changes.

what else?
chemo continues.
lymph nodes swell.
yecht!

posted by Anthony Glass at 9:43 p.m.

. . .

"Your eyes are absolutely beautiful."

"Ahh, shucks." I blinked my eyelashes rapidly. You could still get me to blush.

"So, Valentine's Day. I kinda like the idea of wearing matching jumpsuits and going to the Olive Garden."

"Really?" I was surprised but absolutely loving the ridiculousness of it.

"It's so cheeseball it just might be perfect for us." You loved it, too, but started offering more concrete plans. "Otherwise we could go to a fancy restaurant on the Westside and then maybe a movie."

"Lame," I declared. You smiled at me.

"Stay in bed and snugglespoonkisskissspoon?"

I snorted when I laughed. "Hmmm. Not a bad idea, but we can add that to the jumpsuit plan?"

"Let's see... We could get in the truck, drive up the coast, and have a picnic in the Cruiser?"

"That sounds beautiful, but let's do that the day after." I settled into the overstuffed couch, pulled the quilt over both our laps, and savored the moment.

"Ooor, we could stay in the gray zone and not celebrate?"

"No way!" I hit you with a pillow. "We have to celebrate. It's our year anniversary."

"Whatever we decide to do," you said, pulling me closer with the blanket, "I'm glad we are doing it together."

"Okay. Jumpsuits and Olive Garden. Sounds like we need to go shopping."

"Get over here and cuddle me."

...

From: stepfather

To: anthonyglass@gmail.com
chasityrae@gmail.com

Sent: Tuesday, February 14, 11:50 a.m.

Subject: Happy Valentine

Hi, lovebirds. I hope you have a great Valentine's Day. Your mother and I will have a quiet dinner at home, but we have been out a lot and it will feel good to have quiet time together. We are also looking forward to our week of meetings and skiing in Colorado. We have both been going in emergency gear for several weeks, and the sunshine and fresh air will be wonderful.

We think of you often, and you are in our prayers every evening as we start dinner. My dream is that spring and then summer will come, your chemo will be over, and you both can join us in Maine for some time by the lake: swimming, sailing, water skiing, paddling the new kayaks, dinners on the deck, watching sunsets, fires some mornings to take off the chill, long walks, quiet conversation. Sounds pretty good, doesn't it. Consider it a date. Meanwhile, here's another tele-hug.

We love you. I love you.
Dad

It's just like the present to show up on Valentine's Day. I want to write about Valentine's Day, I do. I want to describe our matching red jumpsuits or the three-hour line at the Olive Garden. I want to write about the unlimited soup and salad, the overworked waitress, the coffee's bitter aftertaste. I want to write that we never stopped kissing, never stopped laughing, never stop loving. Instead I suffer waves of overwhelming emotion that paralyze my ability to select words and simply tell the story, caught in the moment of Valentine's Day. The faulty camera of my mind took a single picture of that scene, that day. It has become frozen within me. Stuck in that photograph, of me listening to a message you left on my voicemail, dressed in a red jumpsuit. Yet the news always comes unexpectedly, even when you're waiting for it. Fear that eats away at your bones, screaming every step just to stay here in the present and enjoy Valentine's

Day. There was a pain in my heart and it was with me all day. I pressed save, and then listened to the message again before calling you back.

chapter thirty-four

don't let it bring you down

My first thought after we hugged in the stairwell was, "We fit together perfectly." And, when I lay beside you for the first time, I told you that.

I long to kidnap our first moments and bury them in the backyard, next to our veggie rainbow, just like we planned. I dreamt of capturing the scent of my birthday in a jar: the moon fell, my skin sleepy. Your hand went up my pajamas for the first time and unbuttoned me from the inside out. My stomach jumped at the touch of your cool fingers pressing my shoulders to lie back, my heart racing as you guided my body onto the bed. I remember wishing I had put away the unfolded laundry piled beneath us. Do you remember? How we couldn't sleep that night? How your heart was beating so hard I didn't have to be close to feel it? I remember our hands clenching tighter. Our bodies pressed closer and our breath became hotter. How exciting it was to fall in love with you, babe.

I wished on the stars to take us away, anywhere, so I could live in that moment forever. It was all so easy then. Is this what happens to grownups? Are all of these moments just preparation for the reality of life and death, love and loss, hope and regret, cure and cancer? I wanted to go back to Shuggie Otis and Bette and Joan and noteworthy birthdays and trips to Mexico and stairwell rendezvous.

...

From: anthonyglass@gmail.com
To: chasityrae@gmail.com
Sent: Thursday, February 16, 8:16 p.m.
Subject: literal

i've been looking through my music,
trying to find something to send.
forgive me if this is a smidge literal.

my insides are fire. burning. exploding.
my skin is cold, ice. trying to compensate.
trying to find balance.
breathing.
this is fucking hard.
and i haven't even heard yet...

when i was talking to my mom yesterday,
i told her that i know it's going to be a fight,

don't let it bring you down

it's just a matter of knowing what i'm up against.
i'm going to do this.
if it burns my hair,
if it has to come out my mouth, my ass,
it's coming out.
i'm going to kick this thing in the fucking balls.
hard.

i was thinking recently about all the cheesy television dramas
when somebody is in the hospital, on the verge of dying.
the doctor always says to the family/friend/wife
"he's going to make it. he's a fighter."
it crossed my mind, because i wondered
if that was my fate, what would they say about me?
"uh... he pussed out. sorry."

but right now, thinking about it.
there's no way.
no fucking way.
i'm fighting.
whoever it's with.

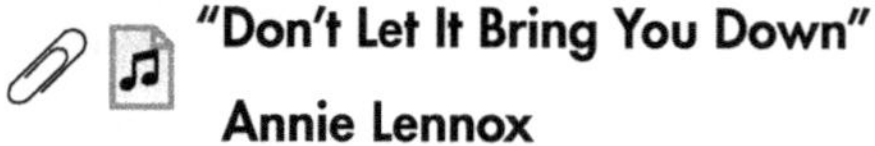

"Don't Let It Bring You Down"
Annie Lennox

even if i am.

From: chasityrae@gmail.com

To: anthonyglass@gmail.com

Sent: Thursday, February 16, 8:32 p.m.

Subject: Re: literal

you are gonna kick its ass
double elbows and throw down…
and it's gonna run out of your body
it'll be so scared of your strength.

I know this.
I believe this.

and sure there will be a fight,
there will be moments
it fights back,
moments it hurts,
and moments it intimidates
and discourages any strength you have…

but you will come back stronger.
you might have to listen to "eye of the tiger"
to muster the strength.

but you will come back to fight,
because there is NO stronger person than you!

BRING IT ON!

and while you watch those cheesy television dramas
when somebody is in the hospital, on the verge of dying,
and the doctor says to the family/friend/wife,
"he's going to make it, he's a fighter,"

our response will be...
of course he's gonna make it!

...

It wasn't even three months since we set off on our idealistic trip into a cancer-free relationship around your troubled and transitioning body. Now, my heart was in tatters—stretched to bloated, then diminished and re-inflated so many times that it physically hurt.

I didn't think cancer would come back. I thought this year would be different. Perplexed and fearful, I tried to consider this my force-fed growth period. My steep learning curve to weathered maturity. It would only make our love stronger in the end. My mom told me once, "God never gives you anything you can't..."

Who am I kidding? Fuck. Cancer, again?

even if i am.

. . .

From: anthonyglass@gmail.com
To: chasityrae@gmail.com
Sent: Friday, February 17, 1:10 p.m.
Subject: Re: literal

here's the new stuff:
avastin and cpt-11

starting my quest for info.
i love you.

From: chasityrae@gmail.com
To: anthonyglass@gmail.com
Sent: Friday, February 17, 3:22 p.m.
Subject: Re: literal

sounds like quite the quest.
try to take some time to relax, too.
take nap.
go for a walk.
clear your head.
if you need anything, call.

I love you more.

There's a non-profit organization called the F*?! Cancer Foundation. They have these great t-shirts and charity dinners and a blog. The website is a bit too punk rock for my liking, but I was feeling angry. I think I passed the denial phase and moved straight into anger. I didn't even know what the next phase of grief was, but I knew already, it was gonna suck. I read another cancer patient's personal website. The empathy I felt for the stranger's confusion and pain became the basis of an immediate bond. I half-considered reaching out, for your sake, or maybe mine—to write her a letter confirming her sentiments. There is also a jewelry designer named Susan who created these beautiful sterling silver bracelets that read "fuck cancer." I kind of want one. They're pretty, elegant even.

How did I find the bracelets? I Googled "fuck cancer."

. . .

–Forwarded Message to chasityrae@gmail.com

From: mother

To: anthonyglass@gmail.com

Sent: Monday, February 20, 6:00 p.m.

Subject: Treatment

I spoke with our chief oncologist here at my hospital. He said you are on track with your new treatment! Go for it! I'll be thinking about you, especially tomorrow.

even if i am.

—Forwarded Message to chasityrae@gmail.com
From: anthonyglass@gmail.com
To: mother
Sent: Tuesday, February 21, 11:47 a.m.
Subject: Re: Treatment

chas and i are both reading
"beating cancer with nutrition" by patrick quillin,
and getting a lot out of it in terms of what i eat
and need to eat.
it's been fascinating.

went to see a holistic doctor yesterday
and had a good experience
discussing supplements that i can take to help boost
my immune system both in fighting the cancer
and against the side effects of the chemo. a good resource.

went to a chiropractor in the afternoon,
and he felt more like a salesman than anything else.
we laughed about it on the way home.

today of course, is the new chemo.
chas and i are on our way out the door now.
i will see when the next appointment is,
it might make sense to come out the following weekend
instead of next weekend in order to be here for that.
i'll let you know how today unfolds.

be well.

love,

a.

"I hate tubes."

"Me, too," I confirmed.

"I hate Dr. Apathy."

"Me, too." I snuggled into the crook of your arm, the one not receiving chemo and turning your veins black. I continued my distraction by reading the high-glossed pamphlet Dr. Apathy handed us before walking out. It was more like a magazine: "Coping with Advanced Cancer." I read that chemo kills fast-growing cells, which are often cancer cells. That's its purpose. However, your body has other fast-growing cells that are also affected—in your hair, the lining of your mouth, and digestive tract—stupid pamphlet. I skimmed to the last paragraphs. A living will lets people know what kind of medical care patients want if they are unable to speak for themselves. A will? Are you kidding me? "You don't need to read this. It's stuff we already know. Fuck cancer." I threw the pamphlet on Dr. Apathy's cluttered desk.

I thought we went through treatment smoothly, even the follow-up chemo went well. You kept active, ate healthful food, and spent time cuddling me, laughing with friends, phoning family. So what if you had a backache or two—whatever. We were on the final countdown. I even sang loudly, *it's the final countdown da na na naaaa, da na na na naaaa.* The song always made you roll your eyes, but laugh.

Yet, here we were again, not counting down the last rounds but hoping for a miracle. This bullshit swollen lymph node appeared on your left shoulder and neck, ready to fight back. I didn't know what this new chemo cocktail meant. When Dr. Apathy handed you his wastepaper basket "just in case," what did that mean? Just in case what? We sat, passing time, helpless to do anything but wait, staring at the wastepaper basket.

We made it home, even ate a bit of lunch. But then it happened, the "just in case" he was talking about. First a spell of dizziness. You should have told me you were carsick on the drive home; you seemed so chatty. I handed you two puke pills, but alas, too late. You couldn't take a sip of fluid without vomiting. I was mad—at what, I don't even know. I handed you two more puke pills, as you hugged the toilet. I thought it might help to run a cold washcloth under the faucet. I placed it on the bend of your neck. You didn't thank me, but it seemed to help.

I never told you, but I saw it. I saw it in your movements. The embarkment. The self-defeat. I didn't know what to say, so I just sat there on the edge of the tub. Speechless.

Once the nausea started, it was hard to stop. You had me worried and angry that it was never going to pass. Such a strange combination of feelings. After hours of coughing up anything and everything, your stomach settled enough for you to lie down and take a nap. I thanked God.

"Don't tell my mother. I don't want her to worry."

"I won't." I wanted to, but I never did. Instead I waited to see if things got worse. I lay with you in bed and rubbed your head in my lap.

"Mm, that feels sooo good."

The next few days weren't as miserable. At least you were able to keep some food down. The nastiest side effect was serious constipation. You kept taking a natural laxative, which worked occasionally. You often overdosed, and then resorted to plain old-fashioned charmers like milk of magnesia and Imodium for diarrhea. The ebb and flow of digestion was either runny or rocks. But I will say, even though the side effects sucked, it was something we could manage. Something we could focus on. Surely this time the chemo would work. It had to.

Wednesday, February 22
for fuck's sake

this blog began shortly after i started fighting cancer,
as a place to inform family and friends,
as a rug where i could sweep up my mess,
and an outlet, as i fought.

and so, although i should be calling people on the phone,
and really talking and explaining the news,
this seems like a better place for it:

even if i am.

do you remember what page we were on?
let's see, we had the diagnosis, covered the chemo/radiation,
got through the surgery,
and were dancing through post-surgical chemo,
on our way to candy mutherfucking mountain? right?
detour.

a few weeks ago i started feeling some swelling
in the lymph nodes
on my left side, between my neck and shoulder.
weird. called my oncologist: "don't worry."
e-mailed my surgeon: "wait and see."
continued with my chemo, returned to see my oncologist
a few weeks later for a standard blood test.
took another look at my neck,
and sent me for a needle biopsy:
cancer cells.
fuck.

underwent a series of scans to see where it was,
and discovered that my cancer has returned,
with a fucking chip on its shoulder.
the cells are highly differentiated,
which means it's a much more aggressive type
than what i was initially diagnosed with.
it has metastasized to my lungs,
and obviously, localized lymph nodes.
fuck.

don't let it bring you down

so here we are. stage 4.
wait a second, how did this happen?
how did we get here all of a sudden?
feels like just a minute ago my biggest concerns
were what to eat for dinner and having clean underwear.
now i'm fighting for my fucking life?
fucking serious?

you know how in every medical drama,
the surgeon comes out of the operating room,
rips the mask off his face, and with a sigh of relief
tells the family, "he's gonna make it. he's a fighter."
i always wondered if i was that guy,
laid out on the table, what would happen?
would i have the fight?
"uh... sorry folks, he just ate it. seems he was a big pussy."

no. this is my fight:
started a new kind of chemo yesterday,
hopefully with better results.
reading literature about cancer nutrition,
fascinating stuff. eating right.
yoga every other day. building the mind–body connection.
started an entire regimen
of immune system building supplements.
(one of them is a powder drink,
and i'll fucking gag if i have to describe it.)

even if i am.

meditation and positive visualization. fruity, but i'll try it.
walks. bike rides. stupid movies.
laughter.
love.

silver linings are lame, but here's mine:
it's been less than a week since this latest chapter unfolded,
but the quality and quantity of love,
of help, and of support i have felt in that time
is something i will never forget.
truly.
i am blessed.
(aw, crap, getting schmaltzy... quit it.)

point is.
this cancer has come back aggressive. nasty.
it hits hard, and so i'm hitting it back. in the balls.
the IV of chemo pumps into my veins,
and thousands of little laser-wielding spacemen
are swimming in my blood, zapping the fucking cancer cells.
i take a bite of broccoli (and all its anti-cancer nutrients)
and i imagine i'm biting cancer in the fucking face.
bending into some impossible yoga pose,
i'm sweating cancer out of my fucking body.
fuck cancer.

leave it to my creative director to give me perspective:
"this cancer is a burglar, he's in your fucking home,

and he wants to kill you. what are you going to do about it?"

I'm going to kick its fucking ass.

posted by Anthony Glass at 7:43 a.m.

chapter thirty-five

don't die before your day

I WAS TOO RATTLED TO ABSORB EXACTLY WHAT IT MEANT. It was a new stage in our relationship, Stage 4. My phone started ringing, the first call of many.

"Hi, it's Julie. How are you doing?" Her voice sounding shaky, but sweet.

Truth was, I was feeling sorry for myself, lonely and empty. "I am good, crazy-busy juggling, but things are good. How are you?" It was easier to be positive.

"We're okay. I read Anthony's blog and I know he and York talked so we are pretty much up to date on the situation. I just wanted to see how YOU are holding up and if there is anything I can do to help. Anything at all?"

The feelings came in waves quite strong and sudden. I swallowed my breathing and my rising heart and tried to become one of those slightly more together types. I lied. "It's definitely been a tough week for all of us, but considering the news, I think I am holding up pretty well."

When people started calling, asking if they could help, there was no right or wrong way to feel or react, but still, something compelled me to try to be hopeful. "Anthony is unbelievably strong and his spirit always amazes me. Not to mention we are surrounded by friends like you, making this situation a much easier one. Thank you for reaching out, and thinking of me… it means a lot to both of us."

…

Paperwork piled to the point of tipping, as I thumbed for the folder I needed, titled *The Devil Wears Prada.* Emily handed me a stack of messages and appointments written on scraps of paper. This is the moment I knew I was in over my head. There were far too many scraps to sort through. Scraps of scraps. Handwriting I could barely read.

"Sorry," she said, her tone sounding a bit like my grandmother's after I spilled milk on her carpet.

Life has a way of being absolutely ridiculous. I was working on a movie staring Meryl Streep. I'd been waiting for this day, proving myself capable of such a high-profile project. Even if I felt I was walking backwards, or spinning circles, I could do this. I could drive this project. It would be brilliant. I started drafting a to-do list. I needed to pack clothes, grab Gladys's food bowls, what else, what else, pay electric bill. I hadn't visited my own home since we got the news. It wasn't your fault—I made the choice to stay with you, babe. Yet, I couldn't remember the last time I slept in my own bed. I'd been warned that the natural response of most caregivers was to put their lives aside. That they tend to focus on the person with cancer. Maybe that's why I wasn't about to surrender and give up on work.

I asked you for cancer cheat sheets. Tacked them to my bulletin board whenever I needed a reminder for the next appointment. Planned my days around chemo, interviewing filmmakers, cat scans, director screenings, biopsies and edits. There would be days missed, but my boss understood the circumstance and helped. How lucky were we to have Kaethy? She was a blessing. She found people to cover my off days. She organized and guided me in the direction I needed to go next. Work was my escape from the pressures of home. I felt like a criminal for having the outlet. Maybe there wasn't enough of me to go around, but I would certainly try. I honestly thought I could tackle if not solve all of our problems by myself. I could take care of the two of us.

...

From: anthonyglass@gmail.com
To: chasityrae@gmail.com
Sent: Thursday, February 23, 12:52 p.m.
Subject: cheat sheet

halfway through the to-do list,
but still need to call kaethy
and work out all that work stuff.

even if i am.

just talked to york, as the word has spread from the blog.
he is concerned, wants to help, but doesn't know what to do.
i told him to keep being himself,
that we should try to get together
for a bike ride sunday afternoon, or at the very least talk.

gladys is sitting next to me
on a giant sunbeam coming in the back door…
i give her two minutes before she passes out.

blazing through my morning.
feeling good.
here's the cheat sheet. let me know if you need anything else.

CHEAT SHEET:

DATES:
july: diagnosed stage 3 colorectal cancer (adenocarcinoma)
august: began daily radiation treatments with chemo (xeloda)
november: surgery (coloanal anastamosis)
january: began post surgical chemo—oxaplatinum iv every three weeks, xeloda, two pills twice a day
february: restaging of cancer. stage 4. began new chemo: avastin and cpt-11

blood type: unknown
wbc count 2/21: 3.6

SUPPLEMENTS:
wholly immune: 1 scoop twice a day after meals
immune support longevity pack: twice a day after meals
vascuzyme: three pills twice a day on an empty stomach
ip-6: one pill twice a day on empty stomach

From: chasityrae@gmail.com
To: anthonyglass@gmail.com
Sent: Thursday, February 23, 12:52 p.m.
Subject: Re: cheat sheet

please include what they removed during surgery.
how many lymph nodes?
maybe call the doctor to get your blood type
and I think you are missing a supplement? ellastic acid?
otherwise looks good! thank you.

glad to hear you are blazing through the morning.
I feel like I just got here.
I am busy. have a producer's meeting now.

will you send me your new favorite theme song?
the one you played for me yesterday?
I miss the shit out of you!

even if i am.

From: anthonyglass@gmail.com
To: chasityrae@gmail.com
Sent: Thursday, February 23, 4:00 p.m.
Subject: Re: cheat sheet

miss the fucking hell out of you.
call me when you go to lunch.

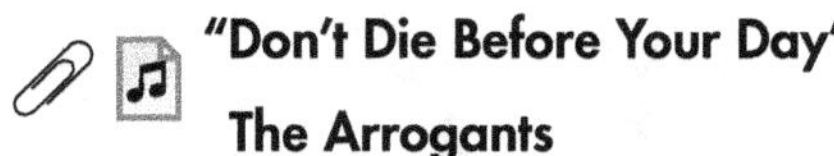

—Forwarded Message to chasityrae@gmail.com
From: anthonyglass@gmail.com
To: mother
stepfather
Sent: Thursday, February 23, 4:19 p.m.
Subject: the latest

hey guys,
wanted to write and give you the latest.
the chemo went fine on tuesday,
feel a little nausea today, but nothing serious.
adjusting to the new supplements, and the new diet.
quite a change to the system, but a good change.

still exploring all options.
on march 2 i will be meeting with the chinese
qi-gong master who's book i read: the healing art of qi-gong.

it sounds fruity, but it should be an interesting session.
researching the simonton cancer center.
there's a session in mid-march chas and i may go to.

creative has been amazing with everything going on,
and i have yet to work out the details, but i am told by chas
that they are planning on keeping me on the payroll.
wow.

chas went into work today,
so gladys and i are hanging out, going for walks,
and barking at dogs that walk by the house…
well, i do most of the barking, i guess,
but things feel good, i feel good,
and hopefully i will be good.

love,
a.

P.S. I attached some photos of us on Valentine's Day.

—Forwarded Message to chasityrae@gmail.com
From: stepfather
To: mother
anthonyglass@gmail.com
Sent: Thursday, February 23, 5:46 p.m.
Subject: Re: the latest

Hi, Anth. Thanks for your cheerful note. I have talked to our senior oncologist, and he thinks your new regimen is excellent. As a backup regimen, if it is possible to be loved into recovery, you are well on the way and the outcome is assured. Gladys alone could probably achieve it, but all of us are pouring out the prayers, loving thoughts, and holding you closely in our arms. It is impossible for me to think of Chas in any other way than as a precious member of our family.

You might be interested that I personally know (though he might not remember me), the researcher who discovered how tumor growth is supported by growth factors which promote capillary circulation. The tumors activate genes which cause the factor to be secreted locally, which increases the blood vessels, which nourish the tumor. Avastin is an antagonist of these blood vessel growth factors, blunting one of the nasty weapons of the cancer. This was a major discovery, for which he might well get the Nobel Prize. He and I were both doing some research at the Bethesda Naval Research Center in the early 1960s.

I am struggling to wind up the whirlwind of church business in order to be away for a week. Tomorrow we pack, Saturday we fly. Your mother will be with you for a few days. Your brother says he would love to come out for a visit if he can get free. Me, too.

Much love,
Dad

...

"I wish you could see us right now. Chas and I are a dynamic duo, running around my house, making calls and lists of food to eat, scheduling supplements, looking up doctors, listening to music, making faces at each other." You stuck your tongue out at me. "It's fucking beautiful. Yeah, she's standing right here. Zach says hi." You started laughing. "He's calling us Chanthony. Anyway man, thank you for your text—the appointment this morning went very well. Chas was there in solid form, cuddling, running for snacks, and again, making faces." You whispered, "I think she's eavesdropping. Do you think we can reschedule for tomorrow night? No girls allowed?"

"Hey, I heard that! Tell Zach he can have you."

Your laugh was big.

"Sorry man, I'll have to check in with the old lady to see if I can get a hall pass first. I'll let you know..."

even if i am.

...

From: chasityrae@gmail.com
To: anthonyglass@gmail.com
Sent: Friday, February 24, 12:31 p.m.
Subject: crabby

might have something to do with getting my period?
or maybe I'm crabby because my boyfriend has cancer?
or I started the day with a flat tire?
or that my landlord is ignoring my phone calls?
or that my neighbors are jerks?
or I have rats in my apartment?
I am just crabby...

other than that, I miss you,
and hate not coming home to you...
hate working... hate working and you not being here!

okay, enough pouting... time to work.

From: anthonyglass@gmail.com
To: chasityrae@gmail.com
Sent: Friday, February 24, 12:38 p.m.
Subject: Re: crappy

i understand completely,
and have had many a morning

when i felt just that way (minus the part about the period).

know that i miss the fuck out of you,
and if i'm going to get a crappy night's sleep,
i might as well do it with you next to me
taking up the vast majority of space on the bed,
rather than by myself.

made my to-do list,
march will be an interesting month.

(huffpuff)
gladys and i were just wrestling
for the heavyweight championship of the world.
i gave her a couple of elbow drops and it was over.
i'd like to thank god, who made this all possible,
uh... my girlfriend for leaving gladys at my house...
and... uh... the wwf for teaching me my dope moves.

besides the wrestling, i have actually been doing stuff.
I talked to kaethy, she wants us to come to cambria
meet her father. he too has cancer.
what you think?

...

I always loved Cambria, California. The town has a charming main street, and a splendid little garden store with a nursery out back. The handful of times I've traveled there I've bought something. Lavender scented soaps, apple seedlings to plant, rubber gardening gloves, loose leaf teas. The aroma filling the store is well worth the six-hour trip, but the garden out back I was most excited to share with you. I knew you'd love it. We could spend Saturday afternoon touring the subtle sages, perfectly placed bird baths, densely clipped oleanders and blooming jasmine. Afterwards we'd eat seafood stew at Brambles and explore the pine-covered hills and rugged shoreline, squinting at the sunset. I had it all planned. I was even eager to meet Kaethy's parents for breakfast.

Kaethy's father, Bob greeted us. His face broke into a wide smile. Giving you a bear hug, he began his chatter of a welcome, mumbling within the embrace. If you ask me, his winsome grin made me wish he was your father and that we could visit him whenever we wanted. His amusing sense of conversation made me like him straightaway. He was the kind of guy who probably knew all the lyrics to James Taylor's "Country Road." He'd never sing along but instead say, "Hell yeah, man, good song," to the radio.

His wife Rose doted. She had eyes that weren't even a color like blue or green or brown. They were clear and clean and captivating. They told only stories of absolute truth. I believed everything she said, and I am pretty sure you did, too.

Bob and Rose were the couple I always wanted to be. The moment I saw them, I knew how much they loved each other. They would do something so indescribably adorable, so subtle—Rose would tuck Bob's hair behind his ear after he adjusted his reading glasses. You and I smiled at each other, delighted to witness such love.

How amazing was that breakfast and her homemade waffles and the fruit plate? I've never seen you eat that much fruit before. The blueberries stained your fingers and the kiwi seeds littered the gaps of your teeth. You looked light-hearted sipping strong coffee and chatting and listening to the stories of Kaethy's childhood; why they moved to Santa Rosa and the Santa Ana Winds over the Valley and how they spent their afternoons gardening and happily doing their grown son's laundry.

Bob, with his courage and confidence, guided the conversation to the reason we were here.

"Kaethy shared with us the news. Stage 4, huh?"

"Yeah."

"Colon?"

"Yeah."

"When did you start the new chemo?"

"It's only been a couple of weeks." You sounded nervous, and I wanted to answer for you. "My mother is coming for the next treatment after her ski trip to Colorado. I'm hoping it doesn't go as bad as the first. I got pretty sick."

"Not surprised." He nodded. "What are you taking?"

"Avastin and CPT-11. The first day was bad, but the rest of the side effects have been rather minor. My biggest thing is keeping up my weight. I dropped five pounds last week as if it were an afterthought. Chas has me drinking these disgusting protein shakes…"

Rose smiles tenderly at Bob and interrupts, "He loves the protein smoothies I make him. Don't you?" She winks at me. Bob rolls his eyes and puffs out his cheeks as if he just threw up in his mouth a little as Rose heads back into the kitchen.

"Chas bought a bunch of Ensure a few weeks ago, and I swear they almost made me poop my pants." We all laugh loudly. "I got two blocks from the house and had to turn around and come home. So disgusting."

"You'll get used to them. Try the vanilla one, on ice."

"I'm gonna need a lot more than ice to keep that down. Though, I don't mind the strawberry one."

Bob says, "Try mixing the chocolate with strawberry."

"Was it hard for you to put weight on while still eating healthy?"

"Of course," he says.

"We've been reading this book about the correlation between nutrition and cancer. It seems utterly obvious but we keep reading it."

"What's it called?"

"*Beating Cancer with Nutrition* by Patrick Qumillan. It's interesting."

"I'm sure we have that book. We've tried everything."

"Yeah?" You sounded surprised. "Us, too."

"Rose even has me sleeping with a healing crystal at night and eating apple seeds for the poison."

You looked at Bob funny.

"I don't know," he shakes his head and does the crazy circle with his index finger around his ear. "I'll try it if it keeps her happy, but you just never know, this disease still might kill me." The room goes quiet, as you and Bob look at each other with understanding only the two of you know. He repeats it, looking you directly in the eyes. "You might die from this. You just never know."

It was the first time I heard the word, die. Maybe I heard it or read it before, but this was the first time I considered it. Death. I got up from the table to see if Rose needed help in the kitchen. I want to be a part of the understanding, what it means to be fighting for your life, but really, I don't understand. Maybe this trip was a bad idea.

chapter thirty-six

how it ends

Monday, February 27
new school

how to beat cancer:
step 1. combine a generous portion of delicious lemon-pledge tasting super immune-building powder supplement with OJ.

step 2. enjoy!

a vanguard approach
in the multi-pronged attack of cancer therapy
is to drink something so putrid and disgusting
that the cancer cells
are fooled into thinking your body has started to decompose,
and they die on contact.
amazing.

even if i am.

i feel it working…

posted by Anthony Glass at 3:43 a.m.

…

Your mom came again with her whirlwind of ideas and solutions. We took notes and nodded and said yes to things to improve your health. I learned how to cook broccoli in the microwave and sweet potatoes. I loved her idea of spending the money to buy a new mattress. Surely that would help your backaches. And yes, I thought getting a second opinion after the next round of chemo was an excellent idea.

That was when she first mentioned a lawsuit. I now understand why she wanted to. Paying for the surgery up front was a lot of money, and what for? To have the cancer return? I honestly didn't think filing a failure to diagnosis suit was such a bad idea.

From: anthonyglass@gmail.com
To: chasityrae@gmail.com
Sent: Monday, February 27, 11:42 a.m.
Subject: something familiar

woke up with the dawn this morning
(and a little bit of parrot screeching)
and felt very, very good.
rested, not sore, just good.

how it ends

sat down with my mom for morning tea
and had a nice long talk about everything.
nutrition, of course, but also jay, you, me, work,
and how maybe we can all fit under this roof.

making breakfast now, amending the to-do list.
the french doors are wide open, and fresh cool air
is slowly breathing in while the rest of the world awakens.

sending you a familiar song.
thanks again for the movie last night,
little miss sunshine.
it was brilliant.

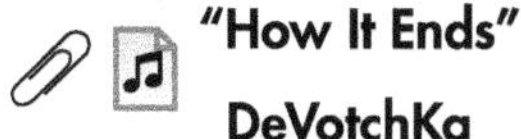
"How It Ends"
DeVotchKa

From: chasityrae@gmail.com
To: anthonyglass@gmail.com
Sent: Monday, February 27, 11:42 a.m.
Subject: Re: something familiar

good song to start the day with.
last night was fun.
I am glad we watched the movie together,
as a family.

I'm curious to hear the details of

your morning conversation with mom,
her thoughts about nutrition,
about Jay,
about me,
about work.

I hope you guys have a wonderful day
filled with love and a new mattress. I can't wait.

I have a somewhat slow day today,
so feel free to call or e-mail me often!

I missed you last night...
it feels much safer
lying next to you.

I was starting to understand your mother's concerns and her ways to help. Okay, maybe my opinion turned after I found out she too thought it was the right idea to live together. And maybe I really liked her after you told me that she thinks I'm great. Who doesn't like someone after they praise you? "I've always admired your mother. What? Don't give me that look."

...

You asked Jay. He said no, just like that. Not a single word more. You told him you needed me here, but I don't think he understood the severity of it. I think he thought of me as a roadblock to your friendship. He might have even hated me. I was always around. Cooking in his kitchen, lounging on his couch, watching his TV. This was his house. You were his best friend. He didn't want to share that with me.

There was another hurdle, too. It was time to tell my parents about our relationship, especially if we were considering living together. I told my mom first. She was easier to win over—as long as I am happy, my mom is happy. My dad, on the other hand, he's a tough nut to crack. In high school I used to say that if I were dating Jesus, my dad would still find faults with him. He'd say, "I don't trust the guy."

I didn't mention to either of them that you had cancer. Instead I told them about your parents, age, where you grew up. I e-mailed them pictures of us on the beach in Cambria, and the one of you and Gladys napping on the couch. I also didn't mention the idea of us living together, not yet. My dad responded in his usual short, cold, all caps (as if he's yelling) e-mail.

Like I said, a tough nut to crack, yet he still calls me darling:

HI DARLING DAUGHTER, THANX FOR THE PICTURES. THE GIRLS IN THE OFFICE THINK ANTHONY IS A HUNK. THEY ALSO THINK GLADYS IS CUTE. I LOVE YOU, DAD

even if i am.

...

From: anthonyglass@gmail.com
To: chasityrae@gmail.com
Sent: Wednesday, March 1, 1:25 p.m.
Subject: rentals

just took a look at westside rentals
and almost got swallowed up by all the listings.
thinking about buying a membership
and seeing where these places actually are.
still need to talk to jay again.

it is easy to get excited about a new place.
a place with you...

From: chasityrae@gmail.com
To: anthonyglass@gmail.com
Sent: Wednesday, March 1, 1:38 p.m.
Subject: Re: rentals

I wonder what jay will say this time around.

I am not looking forward to moving,
but yet I'm sorta excited by the idea.

the good thing is,
we have plenty of time to look,

until we find the perfect place
for both of us, and gladys.

we'll figure it out.

...

"Your back hurts again?" Shaking my head pityingly I said, "Maybe you should try taking a bath?"

"I can't fit into the tub."

"How do you know? When's the last time you took a bath?" I tried to be good-natured about the suggestion. "I'm gonna run one and you're getting in. End of conversation. I promise it'll help."

I ran the hot water with just a splash of cold. You settled into the tub, letting your body adjust to the slowly filling heat. I poured lavender bubble bath, added a little more than necessary so it felt playful and sudsy. You looked boyish as you splashed around arousing the bubbles. By the time I returned with a fluffy towel and washcloth the bathroom floor was soaking wet. You were climbing a mountain of lavender sparkles.

"Okay, you were right." Your eyes shone brightly as I kissed the tip of your nose. "This feels amaaaazing."

Your smile made me want to splash around with you. "If only the tub was big enough for two." I sat on the floor, wet the washcloth and wiped your back.

"Ohhhh, that feels good."

"Is this when I get to say, I told you so?" You wrinkled your nose, then blew a pile of suds flying towards me as I giggled.

"Do you believe in God?" you asked.

"What?" Dumbfounded by your frankness and at a loss on how to answer.

"I don't know, just wondering."

I took a deep breath. "Yes. I do. You?"

"No."

"I can't believe we've never had this conversation before. Really? You don't believe in anything? Something bigger than all of this?" I displayed the bathroom cream tiled walls with a wave of my hand, palm facing up.

"Not at all. I believe you live and you die and that's it."

I was concentrating on what you were saying, waiting for something concrete to come out of your words. This was kind of profound for bathtub conversation. "And that's it? Nothing more?"

"I can't get my head around the idea of grand father figure, a higher power. Seems absurd."

"Maybe that's your problem. Maybe you need to feel Him instead of think Him. Maybe your head is in the way of your heart?"

You smiled, shrugged and paused. "I'm ready to have children."

"Whoa, babe! Where did that come from?" The comment threw a sad switch in me. "Weren't we just talking about God?"

"I was just thinking about the song, 'He's Got the Whole World in His Hands,'" you sang and splashed. "I can see our daughter singing that. I can see her mother teaching her the melody and her singing it out loud, imitating her mother's beautiful voice."

Your lips curled and I saw heaven in the corner of your smile and I just wanted to find my way inside. Be in that vision with you, watching our daughter sing. I choked back tears. "I'm ready to have children whenever you are."

Your eyes started to water. "Our daughter is absolutely beautiful, isn't she?"

"She's the most beautiful girl I've ever seen," I whispered. "She's got your smile."

"I think we should name her Chanthony." We both laughed as I wiped the tears from your cheeks and left a trail of soap suds.

"Uncle Zach would be so proud." My breath was uneven, and I was trying not to have a complete meltdown.

"Maybe we should get through this round of chemo first."

I nodded in agreement.

"Do you think the next treatment will be as bad? Do you think I'll get sick again?"

I mumbled, "God, I hope not."

"Promise me you will be okay without me. Promise me our family will be beautiful. That our children will know the words to 'I've Got the Whole World...'" Just then your shoulders gave and you cried. You cried with your eyes, with your hands, feet, lips, ears, chest, you cried. And I cried right alongside you.

Afraid I might say the words wrong, I hesitated, took a deep breath, wiped the tears from your face with my pruney fingers and swallowed. "You can't die, babe. Because I'm not done loving you."

...

From: anthonyglass@gmail.com
To: chasityrae@gmail.com
Sent: Thursday, March 2, 6:08 p.m.
Subject: miss

jay was on the computer all morning,
cleaning up his pile of papers and getting himself together.
jane came over for lunch, and york showed up, too.
we biked down to the beach, had a great lunch,
and when we got back, Jay's ex-girlfriend's bike
was parked out back.
his door is ominously closed.
meaning i won't get the chance to talk to him.
at least i can get on the computer and write.

doing laundry (separating all your frickin' colors)
and getting ready to go to yoga. yeah, its been a good day.
although i feel like the lymph nodes in my shoulder
are bigger today than they were before,

although i'm probably getting neurotic.

miss you.

...

"I had this dream about you. You were shoveling snow." The voice sifted through weak television speakers. "I... what?" replied Sarah Jessica Parker. "You were just a little girl in a flannel night gown, and you were shoveling snow from the walk in front of our house, and I was the snow. I was the snow. And everywhere it landed and everywhere it covered, you scooped me up with a big red shovel. You scoop me up." My lips tightened at the actor's earnest expressions, and my eyelids blinked at tears. I got up to get a glass of water. I don't think you noticed as you stayed bundled in the Everest of blankets and pillows piled high on the couch.

I stood at the sink drinking my second glass of water. I wasn't even thirsty but the act of drinking washed down my tears. I didn't want to watch the movie, but I promised you it would be a night of snuggling. I jumped back under the afghan. You were thin. Your embrace felt bony.

Ten more minutes and the plot took a horrendous turn. If I had known that the mother would die of cancer, I wouldn't have recommended it. Before I could suggest another movie, I felt you sobbing behind me. Your shoulders were shaking and tears streamed down your thinning face.

even if i am.

I didn't know what to say or how to comfort you. Minutes passed.

"You are my big red shovel. You scoop me up."

I couldn't hold back the tears any longer. They came pouring, splashing with each blink. After a few hard silent minutes you grabbed my cheeks with your wet hands, "You are my big red shovel." I was looking up at you and nodding. "And I hate that I cannot be your big red shovel."

The truth was heavy. I shook my head no.

"I'm not ready to lose you." Your words filled the room.

chapter thirty-seven

orange sky

From: anthonyglass@gmail.com

To: mother

stepfather

chasityrae@gmail.com

Sent: Friday, March 3, 11:51 a.m.

Subject: appointments

hey guys,

so here are my current appointments:

3/6	11:00 a.m.	USC dietician
3/7	9:00 a.m.	oncologist—chemo
3/7	10:00 a.m.	acupuncturist cedars
3/11	10:30 a.m.	eye doctor
3/16	3:30 p.m.	USC oncologist (still on the fence)

even if i am.

3/17	1:45 p.m.	dentist
3/19–24		simonton clinic in mendicino (haven't made plans yet)

the biggest question for me is the usc oncologist.
i was given a rate of $400 for the appointment,
$117 for the facility fee, and anywhere from $0–500
for additional doctors needed to look at slides or scans.
so i'm looking at $500 to $1000 to get in the door
and just sit down with this person and be told
that we're doing everything right.

i could discuss the idea of testing the cancer cells
to find what treatment would be most effective.
seems like something they should already be doing.
i'll bring it up with my oncologist on tuesday.
calling my medical group tomorrow to find out
if there are other oncologists within my network,
but i'm skeptical.

went to see the hong liu, the qi-going master on tuesday,
and despite the seemingly hocus pocus quality of it,
i certainly felt different when i left.
have qi exercises to do and new tea and ginseng supplement
to incorporate into my current batch of treatments.

so that's it from here.
i hope colorado is treating you well,

with long runs and short lift lines.
be well.

From: mother
To: stepfather
anthonyglass@gmail.com
chasityrae@gmail.com
Sent: Friday, March 3, 11:51 a.m.
Subject: Re: appointments

Sounds busy!
I would put the money on the visit to USC Oncologist…

Maybe your stepfather could help think through the questions that might be addressed to the USC oncologist?

I had a wonderful time with you, and Chas.

Two more voicemail messages from your grandmother…
I'll write her this weekend. Maybe you could send her a note.

Have fun with your brothers and friends this weekend.

Love ya,
Mama

"Hope you're feeling better. We can't both be feeling shitty at the same time. That goes against the whole co-patient system, and at least half a dozen metaphysical laws," you claimed, then continued. "I still feel a little shaky. Maybe I need to eat more breakfast."

"Shaky? Yes, eat something. Maybe no more green tea? Might be what's causing the shakes, and diarrhea. Not good." I could barely muster concern, but did my best. "I am knee-deep in work and it's only ten. Wish I could be home in bed."

"Maybe you should've called in sick?"

"I can't afford taking more time off."

"Yeah, I suppose."

"Hey, I was thinking it might be good for your stepfather to come for the next oncology appointment. He'll have prepped notes and questions to ask the doctors that we won't think of. It might be helpful?"

"Not a horrible idea." This bit of conversation was filled with sighs.

"Although, I am tired of visitors. Are you?"

"So tired of out-of-towners. I can't believe my brothers are coming. It'll be great to see them, but I'm exhausted just thinking about it." You puffed a sigh into the speaker of the phone. "I'm tired of appointments, too. Actually, I'm completely sick of appointments."

"No kidding. Me, too."

"Am I really going to the oncologist at USC? Why?"

"Cause it will be good. It's the best care we can get. They did your surgery so they know everything about your case.

Even if they suck, at least it's not Dr. Apathy." I was cautious, but believed my words.

"Wish you were here to kiss." You loathed serious talk sometimes.

...

From: anthonyglass@gmail.com
To: chasityrae@gmail.com
Sent: Friday, March 3, 11:51 a.m.
Subject: breakfast

so what to eat for breakfast?
i need to find some new options
(and something to feed my brothers and his friends),
so i think i'm going to the grocery store this morning.

by the way,
i slept HORRIBLY last night.
yoga is the most likely candidate.
my lower back was sore before i even went to bed.

the boys get in at 5 p.m. (leave sunday at 10 p.m.)
and i'm excited to see them.
i would love for you to come over tonight
and get a chance to meet my brothers
before they have their friends around.
the whole weekend will be quality time, i assure you.

so what are some other breakfast ideas?
all i got are yogurt with berries and flax,
and eggs with spinach and tomatoes.
and i'm tired of them both.
already.
guess i could look in the nutrition book...
but complaining to you seems so much easier...

anyway, big day.
be well.
write/call/talk soon.

From: chasityrae@gmail.com
To: anthonyglass@gmail.com
Sent: Friday, March 3, 1:26 p.m.
Subject: Re: breakfast

well, I have to be honest with you...
I do want to meet your brothers and friends, but I'm not sure I'm up to spending the whole weekend with them. I'd be up for meeting you guys tonight, possibly spending the night... but then go home for the weekend. What do you think?

you really need to take a long, hot bath
to loosen up those muscles.

as for breakfast ideas:

oatmeal
cream of wheat (you loved it when you were in the hospital)
smoothies
fruit with cottage cheese (with flax, of course)
peanut butter and (sugar free) jelly
muffins (I need to bake some)
sugar free whole grain cereals
eggs with just about anything

did you get a chance to talk to Jay?

"I was going to tell you this morning, but you sounded busy."

"What did Jay say?" I was more eager to hear than I would admit to you.

"He said he had thought about it a bunch, and still felt concerned about the space being too small for all of us. I asked what alternatives he had thought of, and he said he thought seriously about moving out, said he couldn't live here with someone else."

"Are you kidding?" I was agitated already.

"I wish. He got all teary-eyed and emotional about the whole thing and talked about how he's feeling un-rooted in life right now, and doesn't really know what the answer is." You gave me a sincere look, asking with your eyes for me to sympathize. "Honestly, I know he's going to come across sounding selfish again, but he seemed sincerely lost, overwhelmed, and struggling."

I tried hard not to roll my eyes.

"I told him the answer to me feeling rooted is to have my girlfriend, my co-patient, living with me. It was my genius idea to then tell him about the conversation you and I had about babies… brilliant, right? Anyway, he starts really crying, and getting to the verge of a breakdown. So I changed the topic to the latest episode of 'Lost' and we slowly pull out of the emotional nosedive we were heading toward." After a moment's pause, you shrugged. "There was no conclusive understanding reached, but if I had to guess, I think we're both moving out—you and I are finding a place together, and he's finding a place alone."

"Really?"

"Sad, right? I don't really understand why he thinks three people in this house is a worse option than pulling the plug on the whole thing. The option does exist for you to move in. But I think the rent is too much for us, and I think we can find something nice for a significantly cheaper price tag."

"Wow. So I guess that's that?" I tried not to sound too smiling. I didn't want to live with Jay, not after all this haggling over and justifying why a person with cancer should be allowed to cohabitate with his 24/7 co-patient girlfriend. It ought to have been obvious.

"I'll talk to him again, after he's thought about it a bit more. Maybe you can be there for the conversation."

"Okay. I'd like that."

"Are you still coming over tonight to meet my brothers and their friends?"

"Of course."

"I understand passing on the rest of the weekend. Plus it'll give me time to spend with them..."

...

They called themselves the gorillas, and your older brother was the troupe leader. He told stories with grunts, roars, growls, whines, chuckles, and hooting. I found it hard to believe you came from the same family. I studied your actions, discovering some similarities. So different in so many ways, yet you were a part of his troupe, too. You assumed your role. Just as you adored your mother, you adored him. He made sure you were safe and cared for. You stayed next to him and chuckled along with his stories, playing poker until dawn.

I petered out after eleven, overwhelmed by the whole gorilla energy. I woke to the sound of the blender making another round of margaritas at four in the morning.

...

From: anthonyglass@gmail.com
To: chasityrae@gmail.com
Sent: Wednesday, March 8, 8:05 p.m.
Subject: a song

this song just came on and reminded me of you...

even if i am.

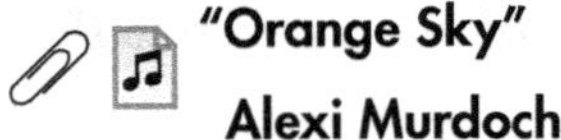

"Orange Sky"
Alexi Murdoch

...

"He had to say yes, you didn't give him much choice," I fumed. "I completely understand if you want to keep living here with Jay. I won't be hurt. Maybe we just keep things the way they are? I am starting to get used to the commute... or else I could look for a place closer to you."

If Jay's attitude had been different, I would have been open to his final decision to let me move in, but I didn't feel welcomed.

Your hands settled on my shoulders as I chopped cucumbers . "Fuck. This started out so simple and now it's a complicated mess. I hear everything you're saying and I understand it. If I was in your position, I'd be saying the same things. I don't know what to do."

"I'm sorry, I don't want to live here—not like this."

"I don't even know how we'd both fit into this tiny room. And what will the landlord say to another person and a dog?" You were thinking out loud, but it only made me feel that the whole plan had been doomed from the start.

"I just don't see this working."

"But hearing Jay willing to try, wanting to make an effort, even if it was forced, it's hard to say no..."

"I don't think it will work." I said the words clearly, as if you weren't hearing me. There was no way it was going to work. I wouldn't let it.

You leaned against the counter so you could look me in the eyes. "I want to live with you. Period. And if it can't be here, then it should be somewhere else. Can we at least a try it here?"

I shrugged my shoulders. "Let's sleep on it," I said, meaning *let's forget it.*

chapter thirty-eight

a song on the radio

From: chasityrae@gmail.com
To: anthonyglass@gmail.com
Sent: Tuesday, March 14, 1:45 p.m.
Subject: forget

sometimes I forget:
I get too overwhelmed with work,
or personal to-do's.

I get so preoccupied by phone calls,
lost in e-mails,
that I forget to listen to a song you sent.

so this morning,
sitting on my desktop was
"Orange Sky."

even if i am.

I shut my door (I should do that more often)
just sat at my desk and listened…

it took me back to the beginning
of our relationship
of sending songs
long e-mails
hopes
fears
dreams,

and it made me realize
that although I tell you every day
I don't think you understand…

just how much
I love you.
just how proud I am
to be a part of you.

every day I am amazed by your strength,
inspired by your courage,
and thankful for your love.

today
tomorrow
and every day…

I LOVE YOU.

I lost myself. I did it with every boyfriend, especially with Five Year. He took little pieces of me, tiny pieces, so small I didn't notice it at first. Until I had a hole in me, this big fat hole of lost-ness, of confusion, of self-obscurity. That's what I do. I intertwine my life with someone else's—much more than necessary, until I blend in like a chameleon. When you asked me to move in, I was standing on my own two feet, not leaning on someone else, not trying to fill shoes, not blending in. I stood my ground, I didn't compromise. And now, we were looking for a place of our own.

...

"Honey."

"Yeah?" I set my earrings on the dresser, turned around.

"I want to introduce an idea to you. Now, just hear me out before you draw any conclusions."

"Um, okay?"

"Don't wash your jeans after wearing them just once, give it a little time. Wear them twice and see how you like it. Honestly, it'll grow on you. I know it'll grow on me because I won't be seeing four pairs of jeans in the laundry every three days."

I took off my jeans and threw them in the hamper. "Now who's wearing the pants in the family?"

You tackled me into bed, howling with laughter.

even if i am.

...

From: anthonyglass@gmail.com
To: mother
stepfather
chasityrae@gmail.com
Sent: Tuesday, March 21, 1:57 p.m.
Subject: update

hello again,

chemo went well.
oncologist wants me to have a scan in ten days.
curious to see how those results come back.
hoping for the best.

called USC to check their availability for appointments.
dr. heinz lenz sees patients on mondays and thursdays,
and is available from april 3rd and later.

hope all is well
love

a.

From: stepfather

To: mother

anthonyglass@gmail.com

chasityrae@gmail.com

Sent: Tuesday, March 21, 1:57 p.m.

Subject: Re: update

Hi, Anth and Chas. Glad things are going well. Next, find the house! It will be so calming and simplifying to have your own place, spare Chas her exhausted, cross-LA commutes, give Gladys company more of the time, and generally bring peace in the kingdom. Might even help you eat better, Anthony.

Regarding the appointments, I have a definite preference for Monday, April 10, for the Lenz appointment. April 3 is the BIG meeting of our Rector Search Committee, to hear and evaluate site visits to the parishes of our final four rector candidates, and decide who to invite to Washington. April 7, Thursday, is my final session of the year with my medical students. I could come out Sunday, April 9, be there for the UCLA appointment Monday, and be there for a lawyer Monday or Tuesday, and then return. We have enough lawyers on the list I sent you that somebody should be available April 10 or 11. The ones in your mother's handwriting at the bottom of the page were cited more than once, and would be the ones I would call first. If you have misplaced the list, let me know and I will send it again.

After Easter, I will have midweek visits with final rector candidates to Washington for three consecutive weeks, two days each: meet whole Search Committee, meet Vestry, meet the Bishop, spouse coming also. Hope the scheduling works for you.

Spring is here in Washington, even though it has been chilly the last few days. The forsythia are strongly blooming, daffodils and crocuses are up, the redbud and plum trees and magnolias are in full bloom. Some cherries in sunny places are beginning to come out. And when you drive past wooded areas, the flash of young, green leaves can be seen. It makes the blood pump a little faster. Soon we will be getting out our bikes and going for rides on the weekend.

Be well. Here's a warm cyber-hug. I hope we can make the schedule work and that I'll be seeing you soon.

Much love,
Dad

Looking for an affordable rental in Venice, California was as painful as a bleeding ulcer. No, make that bubbly, bleeding, heart-wrenching ulcers. It's not my fault you picked one of the most expensive areas in Los Angeles. I still don't understand what was so wrong with living in Hollywood, closer to work—but, it was your choice. You got to decide. I know, I know "the westside is the best side," but it's so expensive. How landlords can charge twenty-six hundred dollars for a one bedroom is beyond me. People even rent airstreams parked in their backyards, converted garages with no bathrooms and bachelors without kitchens.

It was us against dozens of other couples, families, singles—all of California—looking for a cheap, affordable rental in Venice. We became pathetic. We sent pictures of us as a perfect couple with the application. Practically begged to the landlord during each walk through.

We found one. It was ideal, charming, and four blocks from the beach. We imagined our days in the house, cooking dinners in the kitchen, movie nights on the couch under the picture window. Our application, denied. We found another one, equally charming. Imagined our days. Denied. Ulcer. Rented to a couple without a pet. *Damn you, Gladys.* She was getting an ulcer, too. We tried so hard to stay optimistic.

"It wasn't meant to be." Optimism never suited me, though.

Then we found it. Glencoe. It had stencils of fairies on the kitchen cabinets and stenciled ivy over each doorway. When we arrived I went straight to the gardened backyard, stood under the Chinese Elm; Gladys came with and pooped on the grass. Her and I both turned to you. "I think we're home."

even if i am.

—Forwarded Message to chasityrae@gmail.com
From: anthonyglass@gmail.com
To: mother
stepfather
Sent: Tuesday, March 28, 11:27 a.m.
Subject: layer status

hey guys,

yesterday i called the lawyers at the bottom of the list with some small success. mostly they told me my case wasn't the type they normally handled, but i have yet to speak with some of the names, and i did get some clues that this type of case may be an ERISA claim case, in which specific lawyers would be required who handle those types of cases. should get a few more calls back today and will use that information to help figure out where we stand.

therefore, we're still in a holding pattern on deciding when to book the flight and make the appointment at USC. i will write or call later today when i have some more info on that front.

in other news it seems that chas and i may get the house we've been pining over. at first it seemed as if gladys might be the deal-breaker, they had just redone their hardwood floors and didn't want a dog living in the house. after explaining gladys's demeanor, and taking full responsibility for her, and pushing and pushing, they seem to have come around. should get the final word today. if so, we'll be able to move in may 1st, just in time for our visitors.

talk soon.

—Forwarded Message to chasityrae@gmail.com
From: mother
To: anthonyglass@gmail.com
Sent: Tuesday, March 28, 2:45 p.m.
Subject: Re: layer status

When you talk to the lawyers, are you asking for coverage of your surgery? Or are you stating your case regarding failure to diagnose?

Holding my breath about the house!

From: stepfather
To: anthonyglass@gmail.com
chasityrae@gmail.com
Sent: Wednesday, March 29, 6:50 a.m.
Subject: Re: lawyer status

Now that I have had a night's sleep, here's further response to your last e-mail. There are two types of actions that may be getting confused. One is to sue the health plan for costs they should properly pay and have denied. That requires that all regular appeals have been exhausted, and is for the amount of the denied benefits, plus costs. Lawyers make a fee but not a bundle on these, and usually do not take the case on contingency.

The other is to claim malpractice for failure to diagnose. Both the primary physician and the health plan can be named. The amount can be huge (five million). Lawyers typically take these on contingency. They pay all the costs, but if the suit wins, they get a third of the award (a bundle). They don't win them all, but the ones they win make them rich. Records can be obtained by subpoena, and expert witnesses will be required to testify about failure to achieve the standard of medical care. If the defendants are scared, they may settle without a trial. If the lawyer doesn't think the case is strong, he/she generally won't take it. If there is a trial, it is usually with a jury, which is often sympathetic if the patient can show significant injury. A particular doctor needs to be named as having been guilty of the malpractice.

Sorry I didn't lay all this out before. It is so familiar to physicians that it is like explaining how to walk. Good luck. Let me know if you have further questions.

You continue in our thoughts and prayers every day. Right now I am particularly hoping about the house.

Love,
Dad

From: anthonyglass@gmail.com
To: mother
stepfather
chasityrae@gmail.com
Sent: Tuesday, March 29, 3:06 p.m.
Subject: Re: lawyer status

okay, hold on.
first, i am not comfortable filing a million-dollar malpractice lawsuit for a variety of reasons. do we have a case? maybe.
is it where we should be putting our efforts right now? no.
i've got enough on my plate
without adding something that big to it.
in addition to having a distaste for law,
being ignorant of its relation to medicine,
it seems like one huge ball of stress and anxiety
that i would like to avoid.
my priority is getting the money back
that we spent on the surgery
and hospital visit.
this is where i need help.
if there is a place to put your energy,
help me by picking up this torch,
and finding the type of lawyer
who will take that type of case.

i love you both.

even if i am.

talk soon.

...

The air was damp and gray and dreary, June gloom in April. It's tough to stay cheerful in gloomy weather. The Cruiser didn't want to start, too cold out, but the engine finally turned. We didn't say much as a song played on the radio and we merged onto the freeway. Sometimes moments of silence get heavy, for no reason at all. Especially under the circumstances, and on our way to hear the latest test results.

I cast a look over at you, at your thousand-yard stare over the steering wheel. "Hey, babe, what are you thinking?"

"I'm thinking it might be time to ask for help?"

"Yeah?"

"Putting a big legal battle on top of everything else feels like too much for me."

"It's a lot..."

"I feel like my doctors should shoulder some blame, but I don't feel like launching a million-dollar suit against them." You continued thinking out loud. "Is this where I should be putting my energy right now? I want Blue Cross to help pay the money we've spent out of pocket for the surgery, but adding 'talk to lawyers' to my to-do list sucks. Adding it when I don't even understand what I'm talking about sucks even more and feels like a waste of effort."

Little voices in my head were telling me this was a task for your parents. You knew it, too. They should be calling the lawyers—they were the ones wanting to file the suit, after all. I didn't understand why you had to call them, as if you weren't already fighting for your life.

...

Wednesday, April 5

news

listen.

it was a cold and rainy tuesday morning when chas and i
set out across town to see my oncologist, to get the news
from my latest CT scan, and see how this bullshit cancer
was responding to the latest chemo i had started.
the weather wasn't helping our nerves.
does good news come on dreary days like this?
apparently not.

it wasn't good news, and yet it wasn't terrible news.
the cancer is still spreading in my lungs. a little.
i will stop taking the avastin, go to USC immediately,
and discuss some new options
with their oncology department.

it wasn't altogether a surprise. the lymph nodes in my neck
are still swollen, and have become my own informal way of
determining if the treatments i am taking are working or not.

even if i am.

very much looking forward to the day when these fuckers go away.

so here we go again.
setback. regroup. attack.
break down. pick up. breathe.

it's the morning after now, and thankfully, the sun is out.
my list of things to do is long.
it's time to get started.

posted by Anthony Glass at 7:24 a.m.

chapter thirty-nine

vein of stars

From: stepfather
To: mother
anthonyglass@gmail.com
chasityrae@gmail.com
Sent: Friday, April 7, 2:16 p.m.
Subject: Next Week

Your mother and I will be coming for your oncology visit Thursday at 2:00 p.m. and to share a little time with you. We arrive at LAX on Southwest Airlines, at noon on Thursday, and depart at 12:25 p.m. on Saturday. We are eager to see you. Let us know if these arrangements will work.

Much love to you both.
Dad

I couldn't keep up with the changes and progressions and now more visits and appointments. It was all happening so fast. I was counting sleepless nights, trying not to think of dead things and lawyers and a spreading disease. I often thought of meatloaf and mayo. I know, weird. But my Mom makes the best meatloaf, and who doesn't love mayo?

Babe, we spent that night fighting and now I can't even remember what we fought about. I'm sure it had something to do with cancer and the never ending what-if's. The fight wasn't you and it wasn't me. But, I remember both of us tossing and turning, angry in bed. I remember falling asleep with you still talking to me, saying you weren't afraid to die. I didn't want to hear it, I just wanted to sleep. I wanted to sleep through the night, all through my life, though I couldn't fall into it. I had dead things on my mind. Like fallen leaves and wilted flowers and patches of dead grass and the sound of a dead phone and dead ends and dead air and deadlines and road kill. The minute I thought I was past it, it started again. Meat loaf and mayo. Meatloaf and mayo. I wanted to wake you, I wanted to hear you laugh. I don't think I ever loved you more than when you laughed.

...

From: anthonyglass@gmail.com
To: chasityrae@gmail.com
Sent: Monday, April 10, 11:52 a.m.
Subject: yuck

where do i start?
stayed up late because i wasn't tired,
took my supplements somewhere therein,
and proceeded to sleep like crap.

obviously supplements before bed is a big no-no.
all those pills in my stomach, it's no wonder
my body is freaking out trying to digest it all.
no shit, right?

slept reasonably well from 5 a.m. to 8 a.m.
that was nice. jay just took off, leaving his
dishes in the sink, of course, and me shaking my head.
so curious to see how he pollutes his new place.
perhaps he will keep it all immaculate. right.

sending a song i listened to last night.
most of the songs on this album are pretty weird,
but this one stood out as special. enjoy.
getting ready to eat some food, shower and cut my hair.

even if i am.

when i walked out of my bedroom this morning,
i looked to the french doors like i always do
to exchange "good morning" looks with gladys
and was surprised that she wasn't here.
me without my two ladies.

hope you have an amazing morning.
i'm a little jealous of the fact you get to be at work.
i miss being there. my office. editing.
fuck.
need to get that going again...
in good time... first things first...

miss you.

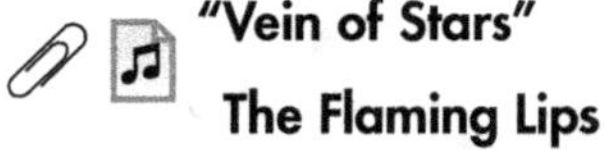

From: chasityrae@gmail.com
To: anthonyglass@gmail.com
Sent: Monday, April 10, 12:37 p.m.
Subject: Re: yuck

being at work is weird yet comfortable.
the coffee is as thick as I remember,
the toilet paper is as(s) scratchy,
the people have familiar faces...

it's like going back to your hometown.

I am already knee-deep in
"hellos" and updates.

I wish I was there.
or you were here.

did we get the house???

sorry you didn't sleep well.
it took me a while to fall asleep, too.
maybe it's time we look into a sleep aid for you?
ok, I'd best get to it. people keep stopping by.

I'll talk to you later
I miss you more...

...

"I can't wait to get into the house, get settled, get things the way we want and live. It's going to be beautiful. You should see the backyard!" Your stepfather was in the passenger seat, and you were gushing nonstop about our new home, smiling at me and your mother in the rearview mirror.

Jose Gonzales performed live on KCRW. His lyrics lingered in the pit of my stomach as his guitar tugged at my heartstring. The music intertwined itself in our complaints of the doctor's demeanor during the first opinion earlier that day.

"He didn't even look over your records before our visit, and then gave us such dismal news..." We all agreed the doctor had absolutely no bedside manners and was a complete ass. He was an easy person to hate.

On our way to a second opinion, we were somewhat giddy. I think it was the idea of moving in together and imagining our new home. We sneaked in grins and rear-view-mirror kisses. Jose was now singing "Crosses." *Don't you know that I'll be around to guide you. Through your weakest moments to leave them behind you.* You had one hand on the steering wheel, the other reached behind the driver's seat to hold mine. I tightened my grasp in yours. I watched the city pass, and the cars and the conversation pass—we'd been here before. *Catch some light and you'll be all right, for now.*

God, it was strange, watching you peel away clothes, settling into a sterile exam table like a specimen under florescent lighting. The room was crammed and crowded. Your parents and I stuffed ourselves in the cornered chairs, merely watching you undress. It was uncomfortable, wasn't it? I'm sorry I subjected you to an endless pep talk as I tied the back of your gown. It made me feel capable, gave me a purpose. Even in my pep talk I couldn't help but snicker at the stupidity of the whole thing. Wondering why we were even here. What could *this* doctor say or do that the others didn't already try? Two opinions in a day. Did we really need more bad news? Your parents kept discussing the first doctor's suggestions of clinical trials and possibly another surgery. I didn't know what a clinical trial was, so I asked. He was agreeable and informed me that clinical trials were studies of new and innovative treatments for cancer. I liked the idea of options. And, that's when she walked into the room. Taline, the nurse practitioner, turned with the word hello then closed the office door behind her. We all greeted her in unison, "Good afternoon." She smiled at our response, her wrinkles curled before her lips. She in a white lab coat, with eyes that sparkled and glittered, she was beautiful. You rubbed your hands together to ease the shake. I noticed. I was sort of jealous, but you looked too cute and shy to tease.

The room's energy shifted as she asked general health questions. You were chatty and flirty, your parents beaming. All of us crowding the tiny exam room. It now seemed bigger with her in it. She had that way about her. She made us feel lighter and thoughtful, we concentrated on her every word. We were impressed with her thorough review of your surgery and treatment. She found discrepancies in the notes and formed opinions about previous treatment regimens. Things we needed to hear to confirm our perspectives of previously crappy care. She checked your blood pressure, heartbeat, temperature, made notes then asked to see the swollen lymph node. It had grown from the size of a pea to a tomato in only three weeks' time. You could see it when she moved your gown to the side; you no longer had to feel for it.

"When did it get so big?" Your mother whispered to me.

even if i am.

With a blink of an eye Dr. Heinz Lenz came in, much like that of the animated Tasmanian Devil. In a flurry of wind and handshakes he introduced himself. He went right up to you. Grabbed your knees and looked you directly in the eyes. Close. A close talker. You shifted, awkwardly inching back.

"Let's do this. Let's beat this cancer," he said.

He had all of us on our feet, cheering. Your stepfather beaming with relief.

...

Friday, April 14
it gets better

enough bad news.
it's time for some good.

granted, it has to be looked at carefully,
like those weird images they used to sell on campus,
where if you stare at it long enough, or from the right angle
you see a hidden image of the space shuttle or something...

right.
so here it is: superman is alive.
he is living and breathing and living in los angeles.
admittedly, he does come in the odd package
of an overly excited,

relatively short, middle-aged german oncologist
at USC's norris cancer treatment center.
his name is dr. heinz lenz, and he is my hero.

going into the appointment, i felt a sense of dread.
i was ready to be underwhelmed by someone like "apathy,"
and given some half-hearted experimental trial
with a shrug of the shoulders and a pat on the back.
instead, i was given hope.
and it was a welcome change.

he was intense.
he was passionate.
he was almost impossible to keep up with,
and i think he's completely fucking nuts.
i'm in.

i go back to USC next week for some tests
and will begin treatments shortly thereafter.
superman, let's fly.

posted by Anthony Glass at 11:22 p.m.

chapter forty

theme song from the x-files

Most of my co-patient routine involved hospital reception areas. Blood Draw was the worst wait. Small and crammed, with a window and a woman peering through, staring, kinda like the nurse's station in high school. I use to skip class faking sick and lie on the cot until the period was over. I figured that's what you did after the nurse called your name and you'd disappear behind a door. Jealous you got to skip third-period Blood Draw.

I read one of the dozen brochures lined against the reception wall. Today's glossy choice: *Loving Someone with Advanced Cancer.* A brochure condensed into a fifteen-minute skim-through. You appeared just as I turned the last page. You had a cotton ball taped to your arm and a piece of paper complete with numbers and markers and counts that only Superman could decode.

Sipping the last sludgy inch of the hospital coffee gave me the kick I needed as we headed to the Outpatient Clinic and the last stop of our day. This part of the building wasn't much different from the rest. It still had the uniform gray-, green-, and tan-striped carpet, same rows of chairs covered in patterned cloth. The same plants and lamps and smell of Purell mixed with piss, bleach and sickness, creating the usual hospital odor that stuck to your clothes and in your hair. Yet, this side of the hospital was slightly different. It was open. There were couches that matched the chairs. Gossip magazines and trades, news, sports, even novels to read. Meals were eaten in these chairs. I snacked on vending machine treats. The lobby was large and triangle shaped. The tip was the hallway to Superman and his staff. One side of the triangle was a window overlooking construction of a new cancer research center. There was fresh coffee and tea in another corner, and a flat screen featuring daytime television in the other. We'd spend hours in this room waiting, or at least what felt like hours. We'd sit. And sit. And sit. I'd read first chapters or finish books. I'd stretch out on the couch, head in your lap and nap. We'd take turns napping. The lobby could easily seat fifty. In the lobby, women snuggled close to their spouses for comfort, children played on the floor as mother and father talked seriously. A girl about twenty seemed to have the same routine we did, sat in her wheelchair, nodding a hello for the third time that day. Whole stories played out on the faces of each patient, family member, and friend. I wanted to hear their stories, but I kept to myself. You did, too.

"Anthony Glass."

Taline would call a name to the reception crowd. The room went silent as we all watched the patient stand, then walk to the tip of the triangle. Once beyond the doors, activity continued. We all knew what happened behind those doors. You'd get next week's chemo schedule and the test results from your last scan.

She would greet you, discuss the week's progress, new ailments, problems. She'd poke and prod, listen and light ears, nose, mouth. After a few minutes Superman would fly in, his hopefully optimistic, charismatic self with such energy and excitement that he had us loving him wholeheartedly. Much like an uncle, the kind who kept a clutter of dusty sports memorabilia on his shelves. Only Superman's weren't dusty or sporty; they were plastic organs.

With Superman and his staff we knew we had the best care possible. We couldn't lose. "This new chemo has a foolish side effect. Acne. But it's good!" he declared jovially, in his thick German accent. "Statistics show if you are getting pimples it's working!"

...

Sunday, May 7
31 going on 13

do you remember your first pimple?
i do.

even if i am.

i had just started seventh grade,
my first year of junior high school,
and along with my newly acquired braces,
glasses, and lack of self-esteem
came my very first pimple.
like many symptoms of puberty,
it comes with a hidden sense of pride
in feeling like you're growing up,
and now experiencing things you've
only heard about through others.
however, that sense of pride is usually
eclipsed within seconds by the greater concern of:
"okay… so what the fuck am i going to do
about this thing on my face?"

thirty-one years of age now.
older. wiser. stronger.
and over the last five months of chemo,
i've experienced some unpleasant side effects:
diarrhea, nausea, farts, fatigue, penile enlargement…
(yeah, okay. fine…)
but on monday, i started a new type of chemo (erbitux)
which brings a new, and somewhat nostalgic side effect
back into the fold: acne.

fun, right?
but not only that, the oncologists want me to break out.
if my body exhibits a strong reaction of acne,

then it means that i'm responding to the erbitux
and that the chemo is actually doing its job
of turning me back into a thirteen year old...
hooray.

so here we are,
almost a week into it,
and my forehead looks like it's
slowly morphing into that of a klingon.
and i'm happy.
sort of.
except now, again, i have to wonder,
"what the fuck am i going to do
about this shit all over my face..."

Posted by Anthony Glass 7:38 a.m.

...

Waiting for the elevator to open, Taline passed hurrying to her next appointment. She smiled at us, then suddenly stopped and turned around. "Anthony?"

"Hi, Taline. How are you?"

"How long has your skin looked like this?" She didn't have time for hello.

"A few days now. Exciting right? Who knew getting zits could be this exciting." We both smiled.

"Where are you headed now?"

"We just got done with Blood Draw. Time for chemo."

"I think you need to see the doctor first. He needs to examine your skin."

We were both beaming, proud that the doctor would want to see the progress of your skin. You reached for my hand.

"Really? We're not scheduled to see—"

Her response interrupts, "Anthony, whenever your symptoms are this severe, you need to call us." The entire sentence full of impatience and efficiency. She looked worried.

I stayed composed, though my heart stumbled.

...

Wednesday, May 17
under my skin

mmmkay...
hmmm.
yes, i see.

so, perhaps "acne" was a bit of an understatement.
my face, my neck, my ears, my chest, my back
have been blanketed with a lovely corvette red
rash-like coating and "countless" tiny fucking pimples.

no, junior high was never quite like this.
let's... yes, let's say its a little more like

theme song from the x-files

an episode of the x-files. a bad episode.

after a week of trying every over-the-counter
cream/lotion/elixir/salve/bathtreatment/magicalspell
that we could come up with, chas and i found ourselves
back on the oncologist's office on monday
ready to get another dose of erbitux.

taline, the nurse practitioner for my oncologist
passed me in the hallway, took one long look,
smiled, and said "you're not getting chemo today."

whisked into the crazy german's office,
he and she both took turns marveling at the extent
of my freakish skin, especially the area on my back
where i had been treated with radiation,
and consequently had no rash or acne.
"fascinating!" he shouted through his thick accent.

this is interesting stuff.
seems they might write something up about it.
publish it.
funny how things turn out, right?

we've gone from junior high
to x-files
to science experiment.

even if i am.

the good news is i got a prescription
for some antibiotics and pimple cream.
it's been two days, and i think i can notice improvement...
or maybe that's just more side effects.

posted by Anthony Glass at 1:43 p.m.

...

"Why are you laughing?"

"To think, we were actually celebrating these zits."

I didn't want to tell you I had a memory of good things before us—that's what made me laugh. About a time when I drank Kool-Aid mixed with whiskey and smoked weed rolled with pieces of brown paper bag. Even in it's teen complications, and erratic hormones, I got zits, but life was good. It's not that life wasn't good now; that's not what I'm saying. Life was just simpler then. When I got a pimple I applied cheap Clearasil in hopes that it would be gone before Friday's sweetheart dance. I certainly never celebrated a zit. This was different. Babe, your pimples weren't pimples. They were cures. They were miracles working. They were little mountains of more time given. We were celebrating a zit as if it were an amazing part of our lives. I applied the prescribed cream, your skin swollen from the breakouts, bumps upon bumps, tender to the touch. They covered every inch of your back, your face, shoulders, arms, even elbows. Your skin was getting worse and worse by the day. *Really?*

Hooray for this? I applied cream to a million red bumps, lovingly. Like it was suntan lotion. I didn't miss a spot. Your whole skin texture was changing into bubbly, deep, toxic acne. I tried to Zen out, back to high school, back to Kool-Aid and whiskey and weed.

"Okay, I think I got it all." I kissed your lips, the only spots without bumps. "I'm gonna be late for work."

...

"I miss you already."

"I'm still in the driveway."

"It's hard to see you go, beautiful, beautiful girl."

"I'll see you soon."

"I'm so happy we moved in together."

"Me too. Now go unpack the boxes in the kitchen."

"Fine. I love you."

"I love you more."

chapter forty-one

everything's not lost

When a relationship is new, you stand together at the edge of heartbreak, not knowing where it is going, unsure of whether or not you really fit together, feeling enraptured one moment and terrified the next. Although you feel like throwing up all the time, you also feel pretty alive. It's exhilarating and also completely nerve-wracking. The possibility of imminent heartbreak really keeps you on your toes.

I understood every word Susan Piver wrote, an instant bond with a self-help book. You'd think I was getting all airy-fairy on you. Next I'd start using crystals and burning incense and chanting, but it was the next paragraph that got me believing:

The more deeply you love, the more closely you feel the possibility of loss. It's really true that loving something or someone dearly is the most vulnerable position you can ever find yourself in. On one hand, you are filled with indescribable joy and gratitude for such incredible good fortune. On the other hand, you could lose it. This is totally true. And P.S. you will, whether by falling out of love, finding a new love, or, of course, by death.

She then writes of her love for her husband and considers that one day one of them will die first, leaving the other behind. Wait, what? Why did I feel the need to read this stupid book again? Why did I think *The Wisdom of a Broken Heart* would be a good read? I am retarded. Clearly. And into self-torture.

The love you so painstakingly searched for will eventually disappear. No matter how carefully and beautifully you build your castle together, one day it will simply wash out to sea.

Good God, that's depressing. Wash out to sea? So in other words, Snow White was wrong? There's no *forever*, no wishing well, no song break. I knew exactly what the author meant by standing on the edge of heartbreak. She didn't believe in words like *forever* or *always* or *evermore*. She didn't sing songs of *someday*. She wasn't a Disney princess. I wonder if her husband had had cancer.

...

From: anthonyglass@gmail.com
To: chasityrae@gmail.com
Sent: Thursday, May 18, 6:15 p.m.
Subject: yum

ate a pb&j, letting it settle before taking a bath.
bath.
yum.
like those.

especially now, looking out the window of our backyard,
sitting in the peace of the house we share,
fighting this insane battle of health, life, care...
so much has changed.
i smile.

i love you so goddamn much.
for where we are, for how far we have come.
for how we never gave up on each other,
for how we somehow made it to this place.
i love you for it, i love you despite it,
i love you with it, and without it.

smile.
smile at all of it.
and then smile again knowing

even if i am.

i am with you. in every way.

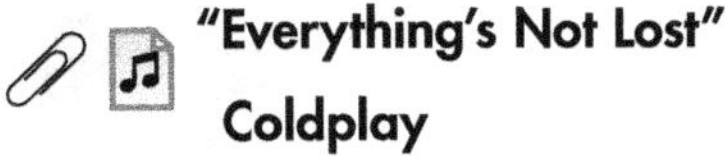

"Everything's Not Lost"
Coldplay

From: chasityrae@gmail.com
To: anthonyglass@gmail.com
Sent: Thursday, May 18, 6:39 p.m.
Subject: Re: yum

thank you...
for reminding me just how sweet you can be.
just how beautiful and moving your e-mails are.
and just how lucky I am.

I love you.
healthy you.
sick you.
beautiful you.

and nothing, even cancer
will change that.

...

I didn't know your parents then. We were merely strangers under stress, trying to care for a shared loved one. I understand that stress now, but I didn't then. I kept thinking; if your parents knew what you were going through, why wouldn't they be here more? It wasn't as if we were keeping it a secret, your health. So, when your stepfather called and started telling me about his busy schedule of summer cello playing and church events, I was irked. Maybe even rude when he then told me about the fine lawyer he was chatting with in Los Angeles who was ready to review our failure to diagnose case.

"The lawyer needs the names of the doctors who Anthony has seen to check for conflicts of interest. He also needs copies of Anthony's health plan contract to see what Anthony's reasonable entitlements are. Chas, can you get me this information, and I'll e-mail it to him?"

Honestly, Anthony, I had this superficial hostility toward them. I know now that this happens in this kind of situation. But, I needed them then. Not when it was convenient in their schedule to visit, but every day—and you needed them. I should have just said it: "I need your help." But, I didn't know how. So instead I said, "Anthony isn't feeling great these days. I can't tell if he's discouraged or fatigued. It's been hard… I think he needs an outsider to talk to. Maybe a therapist. I will try to stay in touch more. Anthony is having a tough time keeping up with all the phone calls. Times are tough, but Anthony seems to be strong and continues to fight best he can."

And in response, your step-dad said, "I am so, so sorry that Anthony is sick, and that he is discouraged. Just know that it goes with the heavy chemo, but should be better after the dose is adjusted. I agree it would help to have an outsider with whom he can talk."

"Yeah... we have good days, and then, absolutely awful ones. Somehow we're staying balanced in between. The hardest part is not being able to be with him throughout the day. He hasn't needed constant care until recently, and it's been difficult to juggle. I find myself tired and at times a bit overwhelmed, but I'm trying to remain strong, too."

"You need to conserve your energy. We send you magical strength pills from the depth of our hearts."

"Thank you." I was ready to hang up the phone.

"We love you both, and think about you all the time. Give Anthony a hug for me, for his mother too. And Gladys, too. We'll call you later in the week."

"I will. It was nice chatting with you, give my love."

...

Monday, June 5
today

mondays.
some of you will roll your eyes when you read this,
but i never really had anything against mondays.
in fact, there was a part of me that kind of
looked forward to them: a new week. beginnings.

when i started chemo at USC, and it was determined

my visits would be weekly, i was asked,
"is monday okay?"
"perfect," i said.

now i'm not sure how many weeks i've been at it over there,
but some things have changed during that time:

1. my skin (see earlier posts)
2. an aversion to needles (huuuhwhabrrrk!)
3. mondays suck.

it's a pavlovian thing, you see.
like a trained dog, my body has come to understand
what it means when i wake up monday morning,
drive to the treatment center,
plug that IV to my arm,
and take it in.
it means yuck.

it means a week of getting your ass kicked all day
by an opponent you can't even see.
it means getting one bite into a delicious meal
and almost throwing up on your friends.
it means tons of sympathy from your friends
and unending pampering from your girlfriend
(but that's not helping the point, so skip that).

coming home after treatment
i tend to feel like a toxic waste mop,

even if i am.

and so, i've decided to do
what any responsible person would do when
their body is filled to the brim
with chemicals and experimental drugs:
write.

i've fallen into the habit of waiting
for something significant, or a scrap
of good news to sit down and blog.
bad habit.

writing heals
and in this case, it also informs.
so, for the sake of my health,
and for the sake of this blog,
mondays are now also for writing.
see you then (and maybe in between).

posted by Anthony Glass at 5:46 p.m.

...

I'd be lying if there weren't moments I begged for reasons not to go to treatment. I wanted to call in sick to you being sick. It's not a matter of the hospital that bothered me; that was something I was getting used to. However, treatment, chemo—that was something I could never get used to.

Recliner after plastic blue recliner separated by a curtain. Every chair out of thirty occupied. It was never quiet at the day hospital. Each chair faced another chair, a twelve-inch television screen suspended inches from patients' thinning faces, distracting them with soap operas and talk shows. Nurses weaving in and out of curtains and thirty blue plastic recliners filled with bodies receiving a concoction of drugs. Some people appeared sick, others became sick. Do you remember the time there was a code blue sitting next to us? Scared the crap out of me. I don't even know what code blue means, but the staff took it very seriously. Curtains were drawn, gasps heard, we never found out the outcome and I was totally okay with that.

The unknown of treatment was frightening. People talked to themselves. Cried. Coughed. Vomited. Pissed. There was hardly any real space in the four feet that separated the blue recliners. I had a difficult time angling myself to hold your hand, kiss you on the forehead or watch TV. You'd wear sweats and button-down flannels. Your body hot, then cold, hot, cold. The nurses were always checking temperatures and blood pressures and changing bags suspended on IV poles. Rummaging through drawers full of tape, needles, tools, gauze. Every time we went to the day hospital a nurse asked if you had a direct line, then poked your bruised arm with another needle.

I don't know if you knew this, but you weren't like the rest of the patients, babe. When all the others were receiving intravenous drugs, distracting themselves with television, you'd happily listen to music, at times singing loud enough for a neighbor to hear. You'd nap through hours of chemo listening to the *Liquid Meditations* CD your mother gave you, but bands like Coldplay and Great Lake Swimmers and The Editors and Clap Your Hands and Say Yeah—those were the ones you'd sing to. Here's what made you stand apart: When you sang, you radiated this warmhearted awareness of something bigger. Something bigger than everything and everyone. Like you knew something the rest of us didn't, a knowing beyond knowing. You could catch it in the way you sung, see it in the corners of your smile. It made me want to climb inside you. Be closer to hear the heartbeat of your truth, hear the music of your divine understanding. I guess looking back on it, it kind of makes sense that you were happy. You understood the beauty of it—that cancer could be a blessing of focused time shared.

There was a kid a few years younger than us who'd pretend he was fishing while getting his latest dose. He'd cast, voicing the twirling noise the line makes, then a splash sound. He'd smile at you with a head nod. He too knew of something bigger, bigger than everything and everyone. He caught a rainbow trout once, four pounds of splashes and noise. You kept singing Coldplay as you handed him the net. "Lights will guide you home. And ignite your bones..." He, too, started singing as you took an imagined photo of his prized catch.

chapter forty-two

house of cards

I HAVE KEPT A SECRET THAT YOU NEED TO KNOW. IT HAPPENED when I was in New York. I wanted to go to New York—that's not the secret, but I'll get to that. Sure, Kaethy imagined it would be hard for me to leave you, but she also felt it was a huge work opportunity. One I shouldn't pass up. I have no idea why interviewing yet another filmmaker and fashion designer in New York meant something to me, maybe it was a way to hold on to my own life, I don't know. Somewhere between cancer and career and life I became this middle-aged woman. After exhaustion called me, after care-giving duties were finished, and after you were fast asleep, I'd go to bed. I'd wake up throughout the night with to-do lists running through my head, with tasks I was certain I forgot. I felt beaten and ragged by Sunday, then started the work week all over. I'm not complaining. It gave me a sense of purpose. But, New York felt spontaneous. It felt strange, wrong even, to escape, but I went. I drafted an e-mail to friends asking for help while I was away. Reassurance I guess.

I started typing:

Dear Friends,

As you all know, Anthony is undergoing a new round of chemo with an oncologist he calls "Superman." What he hasn't told you is that this round of chemo is more intense, with somewhat uncomfortable side effects…

I didn't send the e-mail. Instead, I called my mother. I would fly her out to care for you and help around the house while I'd be in New York. She would drive you to chemo on Monday; I'd be back Wednesday. First, though, I had to tell her you had cancer.

…

From: anthonyglass@gmail.com
To: chasityrae@gmail.com
Sent: Monday, June 5, 8:20 p.m.
Subject: multitasking

no multitasking when i call you at the office.
don't you remember me?
i'm the guy who wants your undivided attention?

just a little sting when we got off,
felt like i was talking to a third of you...
sucked.

missed you today.
hope you get home soon.
love.

From: anthonyglass@gmail.com
To: chasityrae@gmail.com
Sent: Tuesday, June 6, 2:23 p.m.
Subject: i am sorry

for sending you a sour e-mail yesterday.
i know i don't e-mail you as often as i should
so i thought i'd say something nice...
like i think you're amazing
and somehow managing to do so much
at work, here at home, and everywhere in between...
and i love you in each and every one of those moments.

i hope today is going well,
i hope to see you soon,
i hope to give you a big smooch when i do.

love.

...

We go through things. We hold on. We let go. We accept and forgive. We stay still when everything keeps moving. We regret things. We applaud ourselves. We go to New York for opportunities. We stop. We pause. We breathe.

That's what I was doing, breathing. The day I left, I was excited for New York. With my mom now at the house, I didn't feel going to New York was such a bad idea. I relied on my mom. Sure, her chattiness and frivolous conversation could get irritating, but this was her job—making patients feel at ease—and she was good at it. She had an excellent home heath aide resume, the perfect person to trust with your care. You seemed to like her well enough for me to feel comfortable leaving you. After all, I'd be gone only three days.

At the airport my tummy flipped and turned, tossed and gurgled. I assumed it was the overwhelming feeling of driving away in a taxi, leaving you behind, waving on the doorstep. We hadn't spend three days apart, since you were diagnosed. Three days with no Ensure, cotton swabs or butterscotch candies to help with nausea during chemo. Three days of selfish me in New York City, conversing with edgy filmmakers, flashy fashion designers, and then a hit Broadway show. I was feeling a bit nauseated by it all, but chalked it up to excitement.

As I boarded my flight the wave of nausea hit me, again. Hard and sour. I sat down, buckled my seatbelt—window seat always, the middle was empty and a man sat on the aisle. I gave him a quick hello, swallowing the tart taste in my mouth. He wore just enough cologne to remind women of sex and men of competition. He smiled back. The engine started. Another wave of nausea. I grabbed for the paper barf bag and filled it.

"Usually people don't get sick until they're in the air," his English accent teased.

"I am so sorry. Nerves I think." I lied. I'd flown dozens of times. I was sick, legitimately sick, and now I had a five-hour flight with the stomach flu.

The first two hours of the flight weren't too disagreeable as I closed my eyes and took a nap only to wake to more nausea. I filled the bag from the empty seat next to mine. Not discreet and unnoticed. Nope. I threw up loud torturous vomits causing nearby passengers to gag. The handsome man next to me didn't flinch. He handed me his pretzels to soothe my stomach.

"Are you okay?"

"Yeah, food poisoning I think. I'm sooo embarrassed."

"Ahh, don't worry. It happens to the best of us. We're just lucky we aren't flying to New York when it does." I laughed as he handed me the ginger ale he requested from the flight attendant.

...

His name was Chris. We shared a cab ride from the airport to our nearby hotels. He was easy to converse with and even easier to laugh with. I told him all about us, about how we met. I didn't think it would be such a long story, but it was. You know how I can talk too much sometimes, like my mother, especially when I tell a story. Except, it was our story. I can always talk too much about us. It was a long cab ride, and he listened.

I started our story with the comical moments at the office, the romantic ones in your truck. I'd even shared the time you drew a heart in the palm of my hand. Seriously. I told him that one. Secret's out, babe. And yes, I told him how sexy you are. Showed him the picture of us I keep in my wallet.

...

Of course I left some stuff out like the day it rained and you brought me flowers, but I started the story at the beginning. I started it with the usual, "My God, he's hot." It didn't sound the same. I was waiting for you to cut me off in mid-sentence and carry on with the details, so I could finish with a funny one-liner. Admit it. We told stories better together. It wasn't the same telling one without you.

But, something happened when I told the story. I started describing your cancer. Cancer was never a part of our story before, yet here it was. I felt the current of the story pulling me down. Anger had surfaced and somewhere in sharing our love story, I was left with hopeless anticipation to finish the narrative and skip to the good parts, the love parts. It felt as if I was telling someone else's tale. I rolled down the taxi window for air.

"So, tell me about you? Girlfriend?"

"Let's meet up for drinks tomorrow night and I'll tell you all about her."

"I am going to see a Broadway show, but afterward? Is ten too late?"

"I'll see you then. The cab ride is on me."

"Thank you."

"I'm sorry about everything that you are going though…" He leaned over and opened the cab door from the inside.

"Again, thank you."

"Go, get some rest, I'll see you in the lobby at ten."

…

From: anthonyglass@gmail.com

To: chasityrae@gmail.com

Sent: Thursday, June 8, 10:04 a.m.

Subject: busywork

awake, paying bills online and doing other busywork.
(expecting to pass out at any second.)
your mom's taking a shower

to-do list awaits, just as soon as the rest of the world
wakes to meet us... early... Sleepy.

hope you're waking up this morning feeling rested and good,
knowing your work is behind you, and leisure ahead.
i wish i was going to the play with you tonight,
that would be fun.

zach is supposed to be coming over tonight
to watch the first game of the finals.
flaked on york and julie yesterday,
so i'll invite them over also.
wish you were here to enjoy it with us.

enjoy your new york minute.
i'll call you soon.

love.

...

Chris was there promptly at ten, looking pressed and classy and gentlemanly. He gave me a lingering hug then complimented my curves declaring the dress stitched to fit my body. Bashful, but showing my appreciation of kindness, I grinned. We headed to a quiet bar six blocks from my hotel as we teased, over-exaggerating our first impressions—I assumed he was gay in his pale pink v-neck. He guessed I was pregnant with a bastard child and flying to NY to tell the father. We laughed at our pointless first impressions.

I was feeling better. The food poison had run its course and now I was thankful to be showered, refreshed and in New York City. It had been such a long time since I put on a party dress and heels and lipstick and sexy underwear and dangling earrings. I thought about you, Anthony, and I called you right before I left and said my I love you's and described my day. I never told you that I was sick on the flight because I didn't want you to worry. And, I have to be honest, this is the secret I never told you. I didn't tell you that I went out for drinks, or that I met a charming Englishman or that I felt indulgent wearing earrings. I didn't know what to say, so I told you nothing.

...

Chris was blond and foreign, short but built. He was the complete opposite of you. Maybe that was his appeal. His body was filled and full, feeling safe when he hugged me hello. I wondered what his chest would feel like pressed against mine when he lay on top of me. Don't be mad. I thought that. I'm still a girl. I still think things like that, sexy things. I forgot what it was like to be desired, pursued, to feel girly.

Drink after drink turned into late night pizza, and after pizza we walked through the city, laughing loud and languid. I heard about his relationship dramas and heartaches.

He told me about his girlfriend, how they lost a child and struggled to get past the loss. We shared our love for the unrehearsed, unexpected moments in life as we explored the powerful meaning of our hearts and minds. I'm making it sound wordy and romantic, because it was.

He escorted me back to my hotel. My arm slipped into his. When we got to the door, I invited him up to my room. "Do you wanna raid the mini bar with me?" I whispered it in his ear, before I even thought of what I said. He reached for my hand, sex on the tips of our fingers as we hesitated at the elevator door. Both of us restless for feeling something other than our real lives. The elevator doors opened. He squeezed my hand tighter. It was the wrong time to be cheating on you. I know it was a crime and I had absolutely no excuse. I turned to Chris, my losses and gains blurred, the energy of the present moment squeezing my hand—I held my breath as he leaned closer to kiss my lips. I turned my head.

"I can't do this," I said.

He kissed my cheek and the corner of my smile in a breathless exquisite kiss. "I hope someday, someone loves me as much as you love him."

We stood there. We held on. We let go. We said goodbye.

...

"Hey, babe."

"Hey you. It's late."

"I know. I know. I wanted to call… I have something I need to tell you."

"Are you okay? Is everything okay?"

"Yeah." I forgot the words that were in my heart. I wanted to say so much. I wanted to confess everything. "I just wanted to say I miss you. I can't wait to come home."

"I can't wait for you to be home…"

"Okay, go back to bed you sound so sleepy. I love you."

"I love you more. Goodnight, you."

chapter forty-three

no song attached

It all moves so fast eventually, life. For a long time, you wake up to catch the school bus and everything is the same for what feels like a lifetime. It's all the same and then one day you wake and everything is different.

When I got home, I saw the passage of time in the weight you lost, the dark splotches around your eyes, the now jutting cheekbones, the wrinkles gained and the slowness in your pace. Only three days had passed and I could physically see your body's decline.

My mother witnessed it, too. "Does his mother know her son is dying?"

I didn't know how to answer the "dying" question. My mom changed the topic by listing what was in the fridge for dinner. "Spinach and some chicken," she sniffled, holding back tears. She stayed and helped for two more weeks, in time for your mother to arrive for another big test result. In between the change of motherly shifts, we had two nights alone together. Just the two of us, and I was grateful.

...

We made love the night my mom left. Strange that I remember that, but I do. We loved as if it was our first time or our last. We were relaxed on the couch in the comfort of our home, our cozy little home, in the cozy little life we had created together. The life we created for each other. I undressed you slowly, button by button, then tenderly peeled off my own layers. Your movements were timid and weak, unsure of what move to make next. I took the lead, straddled your lap. Your body feeling frail between my thighs, your hold feeble. My hands took hold of your face, my eyes lost in looks as I guided my body over yours gradually, wanting this moment to last as long as possible.

We kissed gently—our breath touched before our lips did. We never closed our eyes, not once. Even in the pleasure we didn't close our eyes, afraid we might miss a minute. That's the way I remember you best, your eyes two inches from mine, your smile blurry. Staring at one another, breathing, knowing without saying, feeling without believing, that our love could last forever. We become one, transfixed, staring contently through a soft moan. I began to cry. My life was right there. Right then and right there nothing else mattered. We understood each other perfectly. We were home.

...

Whenever you would get test results of how your cancer was progressing, your mother would fly into town full of energy and optimism. I'm not gonna lie—her energy was absolutely exhausting. I was thankful, though, too. I could handle your day-to-day calorie counting, pain medications, appointment scheduling, and hand-holding during chemo. Test results were foreign. A language I did not speak. Cancer markers, liver functions, PET, CAT scans. I had no idea what it all meant. When your mother or stepfather came, I felt like a pool shark. You couldn't sink the eight ball, but I knew your mother could. She'd ask the appropriate follow-up questions. We'd win the game.

...

The three of us sat in the waiting room. Your mother typically read a medical journal or medical charts, catching up on her own work. She always wore her game face to the hospital. You and I leaned on each other, held hands, and gossiped about other patients, forever thankful you didn't look "that" sick.

"Anthony Glass?"

We knew the test result routine as we followed Taline into the exam room. I was eager to see if the new chemo was working. *Surely this time.* Taline gave us all a blank stare as we sat in our usual seats, you on the exam table. Her face held tight, holding back the results. She smiled at you, then turned her voice stern. She described the results in medical jargon to your mother. It could have been Italian or Morse Code. I nodded as if I understood her beeps and ticks. You did, too.

She talked for a long while, and you and I continued our nodding. It must have been our naive grins. She repeated herself, this time in basic English.

"Your cancer has spread significantly in your lungs, lymph nodes, bones and now liver. At this time treatment options are more about palliative care, and less of a cure."

Taline's words were simple, concise and sharp. Black and white. Life and death.

...

I used to have this dream. It was more a nightmare. What made the dream most terrifying, what made childhood nights most terrifying, was that it was a recurring dream and I never knew if that night would be the night I had it again.

Describing the nightmare is hard because there are no objects, but only abstract movements associated by feelings mixed with two basic colors: black and white. Jumpy shapes shifting and changing. Now imagine you are standing in static as it envelops your body. It becomes your mind and vision. You become the static. This is where the dream starts and ends, between the movements of black and white, they dance and sway, pair and separate. Static so defined and harsh it terrified me awake, in tears. I would run to my mother's arms for rescue and tell her tales of "TV snow," describing my fears. She never understood my description of the dream and could only console my reactions. "It's gonna be okay dear. Today is a new day."

. . .

I stood there staring at Taline, then at your mother, her face still composed. I felt the black and white motion turning sharp and jagged. Cancer wasn't going away. It wasn't getting better. After Taline left the room your mother and I followed her into the hallway.

"How much time do we have?"

Your mother asked straightforward questions. I liked that about her. She always asked the questions I didn't dare voice.

Taline, choked with tears, applied her game face. Her eyes gave us the news before her words. Static motion filling the space and holes. We all understood the black and white of it. Your mother and I went to see you sitting motionless in the exam room, dazed, simply staring ahead. We said nothing, hugging you at the same time, a three-ringed hug all of us forehead to forehead forming a circle. Surrounding you with as much love as we possibly could. We felt great loss before it was even lost. Felt the black and white of it.

even if i am.

...

From: anthonyglass@gmail.com
To: friends
Sent: Tuesday, June 13, 8:07 a.m.
Subject: hard e-mail

this is a hard e-mail to read
and it's an even harder e-mail to write.

in fact, it shouldn't even be written.
it should be a series of phone calls.
but if that were the case, it would be that much harder.

as many of you know, chas, my mother, and i went
to USC yesterday to get the results of my latest CT scan.
seeing as i have felt increasingly shitty the last few weeks,
it wasn't a surprise to find out the news was bad.
the surprise came in just how bad the news was:

the chemo regimen i have been on didn't work,
as the established cancer cells have grown significantly.
they have also spread dramatically throughout my body.
we're preparing to start a new combination
of experimental therapy,
but the strategy now
is more along the lines of extending the fight,
rather than expecting a recovery.

they told me "months."
"maybe a year."

and so, an e-mail.
after some time to think, to process and plan,
i hope to speak with each of you,
whether that be in person or on the phone.
until then, know that i am finding my peace,
and that as my friends and family,
you are all a part of it.

love,
a.

...

When my mom asked me if your mother knew "her son is dying," I didn't know what to say.

"Mom, he's not going to die."

"Chas, what do you think will happen?"

Hell, I don't know what I thought would happen. I didn't think you would get cancer. I didn't think it would come back, nasty and aggressive, or that at age thirty-one, a person would have to fight for his life against a disease. I didn't think a tumor could grow to the size of a grapefruit on your shoulder, a physical reminder of the cancer inside you. I thought doctors and surgeons and medications and chemo were cures. Now, all I could think was, "What if I'm not cut out for this? What if I can't do this alone.? What if I'm no longer patient enough or stupid enough to deal with this? To deal with watching you die?"

There, I said it. Watch you die. That's what I was doing. Right? Watching. Waiting. I've heard dying isn't easy. That our bodies were built to stay alive with strong heartbeats and keen senses and impeccable immune systems. When the body starts to fail… I'm sorry, I knew you were mad at me. I didn't mean to be scared, but good God, we were given a deadline.

How would God let something like this happen? I prayed almost every day. At first it was to heal you, kill your cancer. When that didn't work, I thought I was being too demanding. So I asked God for the comfort and strength to get through this. Maybe it was a selfish prayer, but it was small enough—yet not once did He answer. I felt completely abandoned. It's a lie, I decided. A barefaced, bullshit lie: God doesn't answer prayers, because there is no God.

I wanted a life with you. A long, happy, boring life—not "maybe" a year. I kept telling myself there was a chance, miracles do happen. I'd be stupid if I gave up on something as important as love. Yet, watching you sleep, I couldn't think of anything else but that I missed you. You were next to me, holding me, but I missed you. I missed watching subtitled movies with you, I missed laughing with you, I missed your cold feet finding mine in the night. I missed your eyes on me in the morning. Your smile before you opened them.

no song attached

You were right there, right then and all I could think about was how much I missed you.

chapter forty-four

hope there's someone

From: mother
To: chasityrae@gmail.com
Sent: Monday, June 19, 2:20 p.m.
Subject: Digestion

Heard the rest of the weekend was not so good. Keep me posted when you can.

I had a thought about his "digestion" (diarrhea + constipation and bloating). GNC has some digestive enzymes (multiple), which I take after every meal, which could really help. He could be intolerant to some of the things he eats or drinks.

I was looking at the calendar and Anthony's chemo. It looks like he has chemo on the 29th and then July 13th. Brothers + friends arrive on 15th. That would mean Maine sometime in between June 30th and July 12th. Did I figure that right?

From: chasityrae@gmail.com
To: mother
Sent: Monday, June 19, 4:28 p.m.
Subject: Re: Digestion

Sunday wasn't too bad, but Saturday was. He ate very little and had a lot of stomach pains. When he did eat he felt better. It was just a bad-feeling day.

Today he is good. He's in the shower and somewhat active. Plus his appetite is back to what it was.

I think it might be a good idea, the digestive enzymes. I'll look at GNC online to see what is available. Also, maybe he should start taking a multivitamin?

the chemo schedule is as follows:
june 22 @ 11 a.m.
july 6 @ 12:30 p.m. (He also sees Dr. Lenz this day.)

But this might ALL change if he is approved for the new chemo.

I think we could go to Maine the 7th through the 15th… or sometime after?

It was nice having you here, and thank you.

I will keep in touch and let you know how he's doing whenever I can.

Take care,
Chas

From: mother
To: chasityrae@gmail.com
Sent: Tuesday, June 20, 8:08 a.m.
Subject: Re: Digestion

I'll stay flexible on the Maine dates. Anthony said the new chemo was approved by his HMO. I guess it then remains to be seen when it becomes available.

It was Vitamin Shoppe MultiEnzymes (my mistake, not GNC). My preferred brand, Enzymall (not the "Super" ones), not always available.

He might also try the heating pad on his stomach for "gas," bloating, etc., on warm, not hot.

Hope you make it through the next two weeks okay.

Your mother and me, we have a complicated relationship, even today. I think I'm a harsh reminder that this all happened, that you got cancer. I remember a time when I wanted to yell at her—shake her straight to understanding. "Your son has goddamned cancer. Don't leave us."

Unlike her, I didn't get to walk away. Every damned day I was faced with cancer, and it's an ugly disease. Cancer has a way of making pain medications work one hour and not the next. It causes intense pain at times, and movement becomes difficult and slow. Cancer gives you backaches and stomachaches, and achy aches. No matter what you cook, even plain microwaved broccoli, cancer steals your appetite. You merely get by on sips and small bites whenever nausea and pain will allow. I had to keep waking you from your pain-medicated sedation and remind you to drink something so at least you weren't dehydrated. Cancer had me applying cream to bed sores. Cancer gives you bed sores. Did you know that? I didn't. I didn't know, but I certainly learned. I had to, because it was my reality now.

...

From: chasityrae@gmail.com
To: mother
Sent: Tuesday, June 20, 3:33 p.m.
Subject: Re: Digestion

The highs and lows of Anthony's health are something he and I have lived with for the past six months. I'm sure we'll make it through the next two weeks. It's an unfortunate routine he and I are all too familiar with. Of course, as he gets weaker (and my work gets busier) it starts to get harder — but we are hanging in there as always.

My mom was GREAT help
(cooking, cleaning, running errands),
though she is not Anthony's mother.

I talked to Anthony about the enzymes and he wasn't a fan of the idea. He feels he is putting too many things in his belly already, and doesn't really like the idea of putting in more. He does think a multivitamin might be beneficial. Maybe we should buy both just in case?

He's sleeping now with the hot pack on his stomach. It seems to be helping. Good idea.

His spirits are low (obviously ever since we got the news). I REALLY think we should start looking into social worker–type outlets for him to vent. Although he shares with you and I some of his feelings, he's keeping a lot inside. Afraid he might hurt or scare us. If we could get someone to come by the house once a week, it might help him feel a little better.

Plus I do think we should start considering hospice.

And finally...
Anthony called Taline again today to confirm his schedule.
Chemo (including the new type) two weeks on, one week off.

The dates are as follows:
June 22nd
July 6th
July 13th.

That is it for now.
I hope you are doing well, and finding your own strength.

Take care and we'll talk soon,
Chas

From: mother
To: chasityrae@gmail.com
Sent: Wednesday, June 21, 1:54 p.m.
Subject: Hospice

I think the idea of a therapy outlet is important. I think someone from St. Augustine (the church just down the street from your house) would be good. If it would help, I can call the rector to explain up front. Does Anthony have any ideas how he would like this to work?

How did you want to proceed with the hospice? Might ask Taline for her suggestion. If we can do that, then they would provide a social worker/therapist to come to the home.

Let me know when you can about Maine. I can take off by the middle of next week because people will be coming back from vacation.

...

Our only task was to keep you comfortable and out of pain. You'd think it would be more manageable than it was. Oxycodone was prescribed, then the Fentanyl patch. The patch was easy, nothing to swallow—we merely had to apply it to a fatty part of your body. There wasn't much fat left, though. I stuck it to your hip and spanked your butt.

We kept a log of pains monitored and lists of timelines and ailments with numbers, scales, descriptions, even smiley or frowning faces. We planned a trip to Maine around pain and appointments. We bought first class tickets and swimsuits and sunscreen. We managed constipation, dry mouth, loss of appetite, sleeplessness. *Glory, Glory Hallelujah*, I'd hum as I applied the patch to your tush. But ahh, the glory of it. My tired heart kissed your pale yellow chest, hoping the Fentanyl patch would make summer go by so slowly.

even if i am.

...

From: anthonyglass@gmail.com
To: mother
chasityrae@gmail.com
Sent: Friday, June 30, 10:01 a.m.
Subject: flooding

has maine been getting as much rain
as the rest of the mid-atlantic?
very very very excited about coming out next week.
hope it's dry enough for us.

thanks for talking to the pain specialist at children's.
it is very helpful to have another perspective,
especially from one that is a specialist.
it seems so obvious that the better the pain is managed,
the better everything else seems to become.
functioning again in a normal capacity
actually becomes an option.
amazing.

the prescription for the new chemo (nexovar) will arrive today,
and so i'm sure conversations will be soon to follow about
side-effects, schedule, etc.
will keep you informed.

still having some trouble staying regular

(without tipping the scales into diarrhea).
chas and i are carefully treading those waters.
fortunately, it seems my bowel cycle
coincides with the world cup,
so when i am doubled over on the sofa
at least there's something to watch on TV!

love you very much.
looking forward to seeing you soon.

chapter forty-five

another day without music

YOUR MOTHER SCHEDULED A WHEELCHAIR TO GET US through airport departures. It was a great idea, but I had to convince you—you were so stubborn. "It's a lot of walking, babe, and with our carry-ons, it could be helpful." I was drained empty from packing and now pictured myself lugging three suitcases and you through the gate. The morning we left I was even a tad jealous as I piled the carry-ons onto your lap and wheeled you around.

I tried my best not to crash into things and people. You kept snickering at my poor steering skills, which made me exaggerate the problem. I turned the metal chair and bulldozed a young man just to hear you laugh and apologize. I was so caught up in hearing you giggle that I didn't notice people were staring. I stuck out my tongue at a little girl who watched us get ushered through security and straight onto the plane like royalty.

even if i am.

Before the plane left the tarmac you got up to use the bathroom. I settled in with books and pills and needed things, close enough to reach. Someone tapped my shoulder. I turned to see an older woman, smiling with kind eyes and wrinkled lips. "God bless you," she whispered. My automatic response was a pleasant, "Thank you. You, too."

You came back down the aisle, your once full frame was weathered and wilted. Your skin was ruddy and pocked, transparent and veiny—that's when I noticed it. That's when the realization set in. When people looked at you, they saw a sick person. This sounds strange, but I never noticed it. You were always *you*. The cancer was a separate something, a way of life that was imposed from the outside, but not written on your body. I knew you were tired, but most days, I never stepped back long enough to evaluate the marks it left. Your eye sockets had sunk deep into your thinning face and your jawbones jutted out. With sense of panic, of embarrassment, I looked around the plane. Passengers looked sad, concerned. A man got up from his chair, put his hand on your shoulder and asked if he could help. You smiled and said, "Thank you, but I think I got it." You walked slow and hunched, pulling at your neck to cover the tumor that collared shirts could no longer hide. I stood up to help you into your seat.

I never looked back at the woman who blessed us but I could feel her praying behind us.

. . .

It had been a couple of weeks since your parents had seen you last. You collapsed into your mother's arms at arrivals. Instantly she scooped you up and supported your every move. I can't imagine what she was going through then. I think so much of her own perspective and direction was considering your seventy-five-year-old stepfather and even her own health concerns. Those are the people who get sick, get cancer. Old people. She was blindsided by your disease and care. You could see it in the way she asked me how to apply ointments to your sores, or her questions about why you kept hiccupping.

"The doctors think it might be a reaction to the pain medication or the new oral chemo—that, or it's likely from pressure on the diaphragm."

I don't think she ever expected her son to get sick, and that she wouldn't be able to heal you with a Band-Aid or cough medicine or a hug. For her sake, you didn't want to be sick. You didn't want her to see you this way. But only two days in Maine and you had worsened, faster than we could track. It felt as if we were running, always running to catch up with the disease. By the time I understood what to do with a new symptom, another appeared, more demanding than the last. Walking up the stairs became almost impossible. Twenty-four steps took twenty-four minutes. Bathing was your only form of relief. Floating reduced the pressure on your lower back. You took two, sometimes three in a day. Baths and naps.

We never really left the cabin in Maine. You wanted to go kayaking and sailing, but you didn't have enough energy to even walk down to the dock. We never went to your favorite restaurant, The Lobster Pound. There was a gradual decrease in your appetite, even though your mother did her damnedest to get you eating something, preferably healthy somethings. She even tried your favorite, peanut butter and jelly. Nothing tasted good. Cravings for pizza and ice cream came and went. Liquids were better than solids. Your stepfather bought some Ensure.

...

Your brothers and family came to spend some time with you. I know it was disappointing that you couldn't do the things you had done every summer since childhood. I surely didn't want to do those things without you. Your stepfather wanted to go hiking, your brother wanted to go antiquing and wine tasting. No and no. That wasn't why I came. I came to vacation with you. To relax with you. If that meant lounging in bed for an entire week, I was all for it. Yet your mother persuaded me to go into town with your brother and his wife. I think it was more for her sake than my own—she wanted some private time with you.

We went out to lunch and took the boat there. It was lovely to get out of the cabin and be on the lake and in the warmth of the sun. I ordered this amazing, creamy clam chowder.

Your brother talked. "My mom really wants Anthony to come home to DC…" I kept eating my chowder, not really listening but wishing you were here to share a bite. "It makes the most sense for him to move to DC. He can live at the house with her, and she can care for him and still work. I'll be a lot closer, too, and can help. Anthony needs to move home to DC. You need to convince him of that."

"I'm sorry, what?" I stared at him confused. "Wait, what? Persuade him to move to DC?" I was no longer hungry. "We need to do a lot of things…" I felt pushed in a corner. I never even thought about moving to DC. It made sense to be closer to family for extra help, but all your doctors were in California, and all your friends. I was there. Why would we move? Because your mother could take care of you? Wasn't I doing that? I wanted to get back to you that very second, get back to the safety of you. I wanted to go home.

…

In bed snuggling with pillows and blankets, I laid my head in your lap and you moved my hair from my face.

"Did your mother talk to you today? About moving to DC?"

"Yeah."

"How do you feel about the idea?" I closed my eyes, braced myself for your answer.

"God, no. Never." I looked up at you.

"Why?"

"All my doctors are in LA, all my friends, and you're there. My life is in Venice. That's my home, with you and Gladys in our house. Moving to DC feels like moving in with my parents, to what? Die? I don't want that. I wouldn't let you quit work to move to DC, and I'm not going there without you. I wouldn't even consider that. There's nothing more to talk about… Why, did my brother talk to you? Did you think I would agree to moving?"

"No. Not for a second." I couldn't help but curl up in your lap. You had this way of always taking care of me.

When your mother asked me again that night, and your brother asked again, I said, "No, Anthony doesn't want to move to DC. I can't convince him." Which was the truth. You had made up your mind.

…

This was one of those tub conversations. Those intimate moments where I'm scrubbing your boney, acne-scarred back and shampooing your thinning hair. Tub conversations replaced our after-sex intimate moments. They were ways in which I could touch you, washing your arm with as much love as the soap would allow. It's when the simplest words and tenderhearted emotions came slipping out in breaths and sighs and sentiments. It's where we talked about dying and death and the afterlife and God and love. We talked about the things that scared you most about death. It wasn't so much the act of it. What scared you most was leaving.

"The idea of dying isn't as scary as much as not being there for my family and friends. I hate not being there for you. I want to carry on this love I feel for you. I want to continue carrying on the life we've been living."

I wanted to say so much, but it hurt to even breathe.

"I think I'd like to be cremated." You'd think I'd flinch at the thought, but it was a discussion we needed to have. One we'd been avoiding. I was thankful I didn't have to ask.

"Yep, cremated. Let's burn the shit out of this cancer." I actually laughed a little. I liked the idea of burning your body. Is that crazy? It tasted like revenge, our way to fight back and win.

"I know where I'd like my ashes spread—"

"Look at me, I need to wash your face." You closed your eyes and leaned forward. I couldn't help but kiss you first, before washing.

"Okay, you fool, where am I going to spread your ashes?" I could feel you smile in my hands. That's what started me crying. It was our fourth night of Maine tubs and the flood gates opened. You started to cry, too, when you told me where you wanted your ashes spread.

"I'm afraid I'm going to die soon. I am dying. I can feel it…"

You looked deep into my eyes, as I looked deep into yours. They were telling me that nothing else mattered. We were a part of each other. Even though we were crying, I wasn't afraid anymore. You smiled as if you achieved what you had come here to do.

I kissed your eyelids. "I love you," I said.

"I love you more."

...

I poured myself a cup of tea and sat with your mother.

"How is he feeling?"

"Tired, but happy to be here. Happy to be with his family, with you."

She smiled softly. "He's never brought a girl to Maine before."

"He hasn't?" I swallowed hard.

"Nope. I think he was waiting for the perfect person to share it with."

I put my face into my hands and started to cry.

Her embrace was strong. "I'm worried that the cancer is winning and the pain he is facing will only get worse," she said with a shaky voice. "I feel pain for the things he feels he's missing. He's not supposed to be doing these things right now. He's got other things he should be doing, other than dealing with cancer. I fear those things the most, the things he is missing." Now we were both crying. "I never thought my baby would get cancer..."

chapter forty-six

transatlanticism

I can't tell you how anyone else feels. But from my point of view as co-patient, cancer is surreal. Waiting at the hospital, I was foggy and confused about why the doctor wanted to admit you. I understood that you lost ten pounds during our trip in Maine. You weren't eating much, so it made sense. But, now they wanted to give you intravenous food and hydration. It was all happening so fast—your body was losing its ability to maintain itself. Your blood pressure was low, your body temperature fluctuated. There was increased perspiration, clamminess. Your skin was turning a pale yellowish color. Your nail beds, hands and feet were bluish and cold. Your breathing became labored, and you hiccupped for hours. Those hiccups drove me crazy. We tried everything to stop them, and without any reason at all, your breathing would become clear and even.

"Hi, it's Chas." I didn't give your mother the chance to say hello. "I'm calling because they want to admit Anthony into the hospital. Things aren't good. I think traveling to Maine was taxing. I think you need to be here. You do need to be here. Anthony needs you here..."

"I'll see if I can get on a flight tomorrow. I call you later."

I called work next, said I wasn't coming back to the office anytime soon.

...

From: stepfather
To: medical director
CC: mother
anthonyglass@gmail.com
chasityrae@gmail.com
Sent: Wednesday, July 16, 11:18 a.m.
Subject: Anthony Glass

Again I write to you about the care of our son, Anthony. Please find my letter attached. The matter is quite urgent, and I would be grateful for a prompt reply.

Many thanks, the Glass family

TO: Medical Director, HMO
DATE: July 16

I am Dr. Avery from Washington, DC, father of Anthony Glass, who has widespread metastasis colorectal cancer. We have spoken and corresponded before about his care. I remind you that as his cancer proved refractory to chemotherapy, and as the oncologist ran out of therapeutic ammunition, you approved moving his care to Dr. Heinz Lenz at the Norris Cancer Center at USC. We believe he has received excellent care there, but unfortunately his cancer has continued to progress.

Anthony now has metastases in his abdomen, his liver, his lungs, his sacrum and his scapula, and a mass the size of a grapefruit in his neck which is compressing his throat. The result is that he has difficulty swallowing and breathing, and his voice is becoming weak and husky. He has lost a lot of weight. His pain is very severe, and adequate pain medication is a major goal of therapy at this time. Thus the issues today are different, and are very urgent.

From the point of view of Anthony, and of our family, he needs short-term admission to the hospital, intravenous hydration and alimentation for a few days, and deep sedation to allow him to lie flat and quiet enough to permit an MRI, to define the anatomy of the large mass in his neck. The object is then to irradiate the neck mass and take the pressure off vital structures in his neck. This is Dr. Lenz's recommendation. He also needs the Fentanyl patches every 48 hours, instead of every 72 hours, as he breaks through and is in agony on the third day. In the longer run, we are planning to organize hospice care in Anthony's home. We do not expect miracles, nor do we want prolonged medical heroics. But Anthony is desperately uncomfortable and deserves the indicated care without being ground up by the medical system.

We have been told that the HMO may not pay for the hospitalization, or the MRI and neck radiation, or the more frequent Fentanyl patches. What is the alternative that is being offered? Is it right that a critically ill patient, a dying patient, should dangle between two medical groups? Is it right that a therapeutic relationship should be severed when it is needed the most? Imagine if Anthony were your son. He is our son.

Many thanks for your attention and consideration. My wife is there with Anthony and Chas, his girlfriend. I would appreciate a call at home, or my cell. I look forward to your reply.

...

Babe, do you remember when you told me about fat love? It was after York and Julie stopped by with a basket full of goodies. Things they personally selected, knowing the treats you'd love like loose leaf tea and chocolate-covered sugar cookies to dip. They knew you preferred green over black teas and the type of raw honey you swore by. When they arrived with a basket in hand, I started the tea kettle.

I remember the two of them telling a story. I don't remember what the story was about, I just remember the way they told it. I remember York starting a serious tale and after five minutes of us nodding and debating, Julie would interrupt with her soft sweet voice, 'No, no. Let me tell you what really happened…" Her sweet demeanor now sure and certain of telling the facts, not fiction, had us in stitches. York wore a delighted smirk as he watched Julie's lips move. He slipped a finger under the edge of her jeans, at her waist, just to touch her skin and be a part of her. His dimples deepened as her story continued. Sipping tea solely in that moment. Watching love perfectly packaged. We said our goodbyes with hugs and kisses and see-you-soons. You said you were so happy to be a part of it.

"A part of what?"

"Fat love."

"What's that?"

"It's when love isn't about the great highs and epic lows and passionate honeymoon phases. It's when love grows fat and healthy and full. When love is as nourishing as a good breakfast. To eat your favorite meal every day and never tire of it. That's fat love. Like chocolate chip cookies and milk. York and Julie are cookies and milk."

"What are we?" I was still smiling from their visit.

"Chocolate cake and ice cream. No question."

I laughed.

"Now get over here and cuddle me already, so I can eat you." You nibbled my bare shoulder.

…

We all felt safe at the hospital. You slept soundly on your back. Intravenous pain medication, morphine… nothing fancy. I liked that it was a drug I had heard of before. I heard that it's potent and powerful. Any drug that lets you rest easy, I liked it.

You were sleeping most of the time now. You were relaxed at the hospital, and I could literally see the stress lift from your shoulders as you rolled lightly from side to side in bed. Your mother and I stayed in your room, trying not to wake you. We played cards, did the crossword puzzle, read books, watched television. We took turns from the hospital to home, trading nights, feeling weak but determined to stay by your side.

I moved outside myself, watching me watch your mother rub your head and stare at the wall-mounted television. I watched myself have a conversation over your sluggish body about picking up dog food for Gladys. I watched myself watch Superman and Taline walk in. They visited every day, sometimes twice a day, to monitor the many numbers and markers and facts. One day turned into two, into four, and then my birthday.

"I heard it's your birthday today," Taline said. "Happy birthday."

"It is. Thank you." You winked at me as Taline wrote down your blood pressure results. You thanked her for remembering. She nodded. My heart sunk and rose to her nods. I needed something to go right. Something to hope for. A birthday gift. I followed her out of the hospital room.

"How much longer do we need to be here?" I asked the back of her head.

Taline gazed past me to your mother standing behind me. She crossed her arms, wringing the skin at her elbows, not sure exactly how to say it. She said each word slowly: "It is time."

I turned to your mother, confused.

"The disease is moving quickly, too quickly. You have maybe a couple of weeks." There was a brick in my throat, too heavy to swallow. "Hospice is a good idea at this point. I think it's time to take him home." She paused. "I'm so sorry." She looked at me, and then quickly turned, crying as she walked off.

I turned back to your mother. She looked right through me, waiting for Taline to turn around. Her mouth opened and she said to no one, "I thought I could fix him. That's what mothers do, they fix their sons. I thought I could fix him and he'd be all better." She looked at me now, unable to hold onto any feelings. None of this was real. I was hugging your mother, but none of it was real. Not my emotions, not this hospital, not your mother, none of it.

I understood your mother more than I ever had. I understood her love, her need to fix you.

"You can't fix him." I hugged her tightly. "I know, because I tried. But you know what we can do? We can keep loving him. We can tell him we love him, and that we're proud of him. We are proud to love him. That we will all be okay. Because we have each other. We're family." Your mother softened in my arms. We continued hugging, taking deep breathes to recover.

Her eyes looked startled. "Should we tell him?"

"No. Let's just go home."

Her hands were on my shoulders, staring back. "Thank you, Chas."

I nodded. "You go ahead. I need a minute first."

Your mother stood at your door for a moment, regaining her composure. I heard her say to you as she entered, "Good morning, sleepyhead. You hungry?" I admired her. I was amazed at her strength and grace. All this time we wanted the same things. We wanted to fix you. I stood there in the hallway, gazing at the chaos and confusion, looking for an answer, leaning on the wall. I slid to the cold tiled floor. I sat on the ground of the busy hospital hugging my knees trying to fuel my thoughts, free my vision of illness, of patterned scrubs, gurneys, clipboards, IV bags; free my eardrums of the noises produced by the nurses and intercoms calling out codes and names and blood and cuts and bruises. I simply sat there talking to God. I doubted him these days, but I prayed anyway, asking him for this test to end. For Superman to come around the corner and tell me Taline is insane, she shouldn't even be working here, she's all wrong. I waited, but Superman never came around the corner. I put my head in my lap and did the only think I knew what to do anymore. I cried.

...

I wish I could've seen Superman's face when you asked if you could take me out to dinner for my birthday that night. I bet he grinned like a father does when his teenage son asks to borrow the car for a date. He agreed to a compromise, a night's walk through the campus gardens. We had a curfew, after which we needed to be back in bed. The doctors unplugged the fluid hydration. We carried only a small pack of pain medication like an old cassette player. You pushed play to receive another dose and joked, "What should we listen to now. A little *Transatlanticism* maybe?"

Even in the July heat you wore a sweater over your hospital gown and a blanket over your legs for warmth. Your mother kissed you good night on the forehead and left for the evening. I nodded at her, remembering what we agreed on. She smiled back knowingly.

I wheeled you to the elevator and ran out the hospital doors. You howled, "Run faster!" The air was warm and soft, the moon shone brightly, lit our path around campus. We found a small park, only the size of a large backyard and lined with buildings and benches. In the center, grass, roses, agapanthus, large liquid ambers, maples and magnolias all in bloom. The air was fragrant and sweet as candy. Night stretched all around us, and bugs flittered in the park lights, dancing with joy. The sky was filled with stars. Everything shined and sparkled and twinkled as I gave you a tour of my hospital and the spots I frequented.

"And here's where I eat lunch when you're at chemo, and over there is…"

"Chas. Can you stop for a minute?"

"Sure." I stood still, locked the wheels of your chair and walked in front to face you. "You okay?"

"Yeah. I just wanted to see you." Your eyes twinkled. "You're beautiful. I know I've told you that 284 times, but I needed to tell you again. I think you're absolutely beautiful."

I knelt on the concrete and kissed you with my nose. "Make that 285 times." I teased tickling your cheek with mine.

"This is a perfect night isn't it?"

I looked around. "You took the words right out of my mouth."

You grabbed my hand and placed it on your cheek. "It's not the night that makes it perfect…" You kissed my palm. Closed your eyes and nuzzled your features in my hand.

"Don't get all sappy on me now." I kissed your cheek softly but firmly, holding back the rising sorrow. "Let's go sit over there. I sometimes take a nap on that bench when you are at the day hospital. It's warm in the sun."

"You do?"

"Yeah."

"I hate the idea of you sleeping on a bench. I hate the idea of you here at all." Babe, I didn't know what you were about to say, but nerves had you looking down. "Chas, I need you to know…" I sat on the bench, spread my legs and pulled your wheelchair in between, leaned forward and kissed the tip of your chin. "I need you to know… I love you."

You snatched my breath. I pressed my cheek again to yours. I got this urge to wheel you the hell out of there. To get you drunk, have my way with you like we used to. I wanted you close enough to take off all your clothes and bite your skin.

I wished that time moved backward. That you were born with cancer and died in the womb. I wished we were there right now playing ring-around-the-rosie. I wished that the wheels spun in reverse. That the earth sucked the tomatoes we planted out of the air, back into their stem pulling them back into a seed of a ripe red tomato. That we were drunk then sober. Had dessert before dinner. That we read last chapters before firsts. That timelines were beginnings and not endings.

"You're the most beautiful, courageous person I know. And everything you've done for me has been remarkable and stunning. I don't tell you often enough, but I think you're amazing and I am thankful for every moment we have together, no matter how beautiful or trivial..." You became speechless and your lack of words wrung tears out of us both.

"I love you more," I managed to say. I wanted to reach into time and go back to the beginning, go back to the copy machine incident. I prayed to God as if I were God. I prayed that my embrace would repair you. Prayed that disease would leave you and enter me. Prayed that I could die for you, or at the very least, die with you. I prayed I too was dying.

I prayed that I was powerful enough to heal you with the words *I love you*, and so I said it again with complete conviction. You answered, "I love you more."

I held your face to mine. I wanted you to see my words. "Babe, I know you love me. But, if there is ever a day I forget, will you come back to remind me?" Your eyes were sleepy, your head heavy. Crying was exhausting.

"Yes. I will always remind you, because I fucking love you." You closed your eyes and took a deep breath, tears streaming down both cheeks.

"I think it's time for us to head back," I said softly.

"No, not yet, fifteen more minutes."

We nuzzled our cheeks and eyes, kissing chins and jawbones and necks. "There is something I need to ask you. But not here. Promise me we'll go out to dinner for your birthday when we get home."

"I promise."

chapter forty-seven

jet engine noises

Your stepfather arrived at our house soon after the news. He set up hospice. Everything was in place by the time we checked out of the hospital. Machines littered our home: oxygen tanks, blood pressure sleeves, stainless steel dishes, trash cans, antibacterial soap, stethoscopes, penlights, digital thermometers, bedpans, commodes. There were nurses, around-the-clock staff, a case manager and a nervous Gladys to welcome us. The nurses wheeled you from the car to the steps of our front door, and when everyone tried to carry you up three stairs, you stopped them. You stood. You wobbled, stared at the stairs and took a deep breath before walking up the steps, through the entrance, and onto the couch. I know it wasn't right to be so proud of you in that moment, but it was all I had.

We assumed our roles as if it was another normal, everyday afternoon. Your mother made up the twin hospital bed installed in our bedroom next to our queen. You turned on the television. Your stepfather started cooking dinner. I fed Gladys. The nurse took your temperature. This didn't feel like home anymore.

...

That night, and every night after, I couldn't sleep. Your bed kept filling with air and slowly releasing it. I swear it was powered by an engine, a loud jet engine flying through our bedroom. I could hear your stepfather snoring in the night, or maybe it was Gladys. I started doing sit-ups in bed, tiring myself out so I could rest. Every sense around me had changed: sight, sound, smell, touch, taste. My blankets were heavy and I was afraid of the dark—afraid that you would abandon me in it. Life has a way of feeling worse in the middle of the night. I held onto the words you spoke earlier: "I don't want you to be alone. If anything should happen to me, I don't want you to be alone."

I wanted to kick your stupid jet engine. *How can you sleep through that noise?* I wanted the warmth of your arm over my shoulders, not this scratchy quilt. You were so far away, miles away. "In another bed" might as well have been another house, another state.

Here's the strange thing, what kept me awake for most of the night—I literally felt you moving closer to heaven. I can't quiet explain it. I just did. I felt you sacrificing life, leaving everything behind. I remember sitting up to examine you, making sure you were still breathing. I watched the transformation of acceptance, of understanding, in the rise and fall of your chest, your half-opened eyes, the curve of your lips in a crescent moon.

"I'll let you hold me if you want to. Do you want to hold me?" You didn't respond. So, I pulled the covers over my head. There was this sense of wonderment at the terrible, grotesque and sublimely beautiful shift that was happening all around me in our bedroom. I decided there was only one thing left worth hoping for. Under the covers I prayed aloud, "If you must take him, Poppy, take him soon, take him now when he's sleeping. Take him with grace, and absolute love."

I inhaled and held my breath to listen. It was quiet, too quiet. I peeked over the edge of the blankets, sat up, looked at you. Panic set in when I didn't see your chest fill. I nervously reached for your hand to see if you were still with me, and checked for a pulse. I see the curve of your lips widen, holding back a smile.

"Tell Poppy I'm not ready to go yet."

I threw a pillow at you, "You're such an asshole."

You laughed. "Go to bed. I can't sleep with you praying so loud..."

I threw another pillow at you.

chapter forty-eight

hold you forever

Loving someone with cancer does strange things to time. It moves so fast and so slow. On one hand, it seems like yesterday that you were helping me load the dishwasher, bending down to hand me glass after glass to return to the cabinet. We were carefree and it felt as if we could live in that moment for a long, long time. And then time quickened: I woke up and, just like that, everything was different. I had to help you dress because you were too weak to do it yourself. We fit each arm in its sleeve, a slow, agonizing process. It fit you differently now; everything had changed, and it seemed unreasonable to me that it was the same shirt.

...

"Whatcha guys talking about?"

Your mother smiled. "Anthony wants to ask you something..."

"Will you have dinner with me tonight?"

"Is that the secret you two have been discussing?" You and your mother said yes in unison.

I'm not sure what made me so nervous. I think it was a mixture of fear and time passing and excitement and wondering why you were having secret conversations with your mother. There was no reason to be anxious about a birthday dinner. Yet, I had this jumpy energy dancing inside. I knew from your stepfather's cooking all afternoon and your mother's detailed decorating of our patio table that this was meant to be a special dinner. I felt even more timid after your mother requested that I wear the sundress you bought me for my birthday.

"He hasn't seen you in it. I think he'd like that very much."

My heartbeat grew louder as I dressed. Your parents made me wait in the bathroom to put the finishing touches on the evening. I could hear dishes rattling in the sink and mumbled conversations. Your stepfather came to the bathroom door and knocked.

"Hello, Miss?"

I opened the door, completely confused.

"Hello. The gentleman you are meeting for dinner tonight is right this way. Sorry to keep you waiting. Did you have a hard time finding the restaurant?" I laughed at how sweet your stepfather looked in his apron as he offered me his arm as an escort to our reserved table.

"Yes, yes. This restaurant was impossible to find." I giggled. "There's not even a sign out front—so like Los Angeles." I blushed when I saw you. "You are a sneaky one aren't you." I shook my head as you stood to kiss me hello.

Your mother approached the table, a towel draped over her arm, offered us a glass of wine. "My name is Nancy, and I'll be your waitress for the evening." Delighted, we grinned at each other as she informed us what was on the menu.

There were flickering candles through our yard and around the patio. As if fireflies were blinking and swaying and flittering. Not the slightest breeze to ruffle a leaf, or sway a strand of hair—only temperature and flickering fireflies of candlelight and stillness. There was music, though. Ray Lamontagne serenaded the moon. *I could hold you in my arms forever.* The melody caressed the moment, following the shape of it.

Your mother returned with plates of food and told us to enjoy. We both glanced at the food, grabbed for our utensils and started eating. You had a few bites, then turned to face me. "I can't eat." You looked down at your food and then back up at me. Puzzled, I put my fork down.

"You're the answer." You paused, then grabbed my hands and held them in your lap. I could feel you shaking. "You are my answer to all the questions I have." You stumbled over your words. "I think a lot of times my relationships were about trying to figure out myself, and the other person in my life—who that's going to be and how they're going to fit… but you, you fit that perfectly."

You leaned into my smile with little whispers and nudges and kisses. The music danced its way into my lungs, filling me with the importance of the moment. You were tender and huggable, squeezing my fingers tight. It was only you, me, and the melody. *I could hold you in my arms forever.* Forever, for us, was right then.

"Chas," you exhaled, "to have you as my wife, if only for a day, means everything to me. Will you marry me?"

chapter forty-nine

church bells

YOUR STEPFATHER CALLED THE EPISCOPAL CHURCH TO ARrange a meeting at our house later that afternoon with Laura, the recommended reverend for the ceremony. Your mother and I planned to shop for wedding rings at the antique jewelry dealer next to the church.

The store was filled with dozens and dozen of antique rings. Each having a past and a story and a love attached to it. I kept wondering how they ended up here. Your mother and I made up stories for each ring we tried on.

I must have scrutinized a hundred, before I picked three. I never thought I'd have a proper wedding ring. I'm one of those girls who likes turquoise or something different. Something unique, not traditional. We never talked about what kind of ring I wanted. I think girls think they aren't the diamond ring types until they put on a diamond. I was a diamond girl. Your mother was busy sharing our love story with the salesclerk, as I kept staring at the diamond on my hand, listening to her version of our love. I have a diamond ring on my finger. I'm engaged. The sales clerk handed us three rings to take home for you to choose which one to place on my finger.

...

"Hello, pleasure to meet you." I shook Laura's hand and stared at the streak of hot pink dye in her short, choppy haircut. She was dressed in a black shirt with a clerical collar and jeans. I thought she looked kind of edgy for clergy. She was round and witty. Your voice was faint, but you had this vitality as you told her about our plans.

"We'd like to get married under the tree." You shuffled to the backyard to show her.

"What a beautiful garden." She scanned the backyard as Gladys nuzzled her head under her hand. Laura scratched her ear. Your mother, stepfather, all of us stood under the elm.

"What days are you available?" Your mother inquired.

"Well, my schedule is rather busy. I do have an opening two weeks from Saturday." We all nodded.

"That would give us a little more time to plan," your mother replied.

Laura watched you contemplating the tree with a grin.

"What are you thinking about, babe?" I asked.

"I think it is going to be an absolutely beautiful wedding. Gladys will be the ring-bearer." She wiggled hearing her name. You reached for my hand to hold it as Gladys stood between us.

Laura contemplated our hands held, then Gladys. She looked back and forth between all of us who were still looking up at a tree. “You know, I could also do it tomorrow. I have the day off…”

Gladys wagged her tail frantically.

“We’d like that.” You responded looking at me, squeezing my hand tighter.

…

“You’re getting married tomorrow!” April, our hospice case manager, hugged me in congratulations. I think hugging was part of her job description and she was very good at her job.

“I know. Crazy right?”

“Not crazy. I think it’s perfect.” She hugged me again. “Since we met, I’ve been thinking of you and Anthony every day. I can’t stop thinking about your love. I’ve been a case manager for hospice for a long, long time and I have never witnessed such love, such sacrifice. You may not believe this, but your love is absolutely inspiring. You are a brave soul, my friend.”

“Thank you.”

“No, I should be thanking you for the honor and opportunity to share in your love and to care for Anthony. My heart goes out to you. He is a remarkable man.”

I looked to the bedroom door you are sleeping behind. "He is, isn't he?"

"And you're a remarkable woman. You carry yourself with such grace and love that I can only offer you tears of absolute joy on your wedding day."

She wept. This time I hugged her.

"Are you going to have a reception?" She wiped away her tears.

"Yeah, maybe. I'd like that."

...

I called my parents that night. I told them about the proposal. I told them about the timeline. I told them I was getting married in the morning. My mom was upset. My dad, confused. Both understood, and both were disappointed they weren't going to be part of my wedding day. It broke my heart, but not nearly as much as it broke theirs.

...

"What did they say?" Your mother asked woefully.

"They're disappointed, but I think they understand the circumstances." I answered directly even though her question made me sad. "I just wish I could share it with my mom. I wish my dad could walk me down the aisle. I guess it's sorta like eloping? I have everything I need right here. As long as Anthony shows up…" We both giggle a little. "I have a favor to ask you."

"Sure."

"What do you think about having a reception tomorrow night? Something small, not too fancy. We could invite people to the house for cake and champagne. It will give Anthony the chance to see his friends. Everyone keeps calling and I know they would like to see him. I'd like to share tomorrow with them. We should celebrate our wedding."

"I think it is a perfect idea. I'll go to the store tonight and get everything we'll need. Maybe we can decorate some, too."

I'm not sure what I would have done without your mother. I reached for her hand and held it. "I'm getting married tomorrow." I said it out loud to believe it.

chapter fifty

daa na na na

ANTICIPATION HAD ME UP EARLIER THAN THE REST OF THE house. I slipped out of bed, tried not to wake you and went directly to the computer.

From: chasityrae@gmail.com
To: friends
Sent: Wednesday, July 26, 8:14 a.m.
Subject: true love

They say true love is unconditional, ours, bittersweet.

On July 23rd, Anthony proposed.
A proposal so sweet, so thoughtful, so pure,
that today, we are getting married
under the tree in our backyard.

even if i am.

"To have you as my wife, even for a day, means everything to me..."

Please join us this evening for our reception to celebrate love, and to celebrate life.

Our house at 6:00 p.m. (It's okay if you're late.)
We will cook dinner on the grill. Have champagne and cake.
Please do not bring anything and dress comfortably.

Our reception is meant only for you to share your love,
and a chance for us to share ours.

I went to the kitchen, your mother greeted me with a coffee and a smile. "Today's the big day. You want to help me decorate? We don't have much time..." I grabbed the ribbons, ran giddily into the backyard, Gladys chasing after me. Still in my pajamas I hung white ribbons from the tree branches, low and streaming. Your mother pointed to places I missed as she decorated the chairs for us with white ribbons and flowers from our garden. It looked like *A Midsummer's Night's Dream* and that fairies might appear during the ceremony. It was a beautiful, perfect July day. Not a cloud in the sky. While I hung the ribbons, "Let Myself Fall" hummed in my ears; *I let myself fall in love with you. There was no turning back since I let myself fall in love with you.*

...

"Wake up, my fiancé."

You puckered your lips for a kiss before opening your eyes. "We're getting married today." You sat up in bed, stretched your arms wide. "Will you ask the nurse to come in? I'm ready to stop the pain medication. Let's unplug me already."

It was something you requested with April the day before. You wanted to be absolutely present during the ceremony, without machines that would get in the way of your vows. Everyone, hospice, the doctors, your parents—we all agreed.

"Are you sure?"

"Yeah. I don't want to miss a thing today."

I jumped on your bed and kissed you as you bounced. "I'll go get her, but think about what you want to wear to your wedding."

"What are you gonna wear?"

I blushed. "I have no idea..."

...

You were so funny. Do you remember how long it took for you to pick out what you were going to wear? I think you did that on purpose. You knew exactly what you wanted to put on; you just liked me holding up each shirt asking, "How about this one?" You decided on pants, the ones you wore to your brother's wedding. If time would have allowed him to be here, he would have been your best man. The black tuxedo pants from his wedding would have to do. Crisp, ironed, and already perfect. For shirts you had a handful of options. From white, to colors, striped to pattern. In all of your choosing, you picked out a light (almost white, but not quite) pink linen shirt, declaring, "I can't wear white on my wedding day."

It still makes me laugh.

Getting ready without pain medication took enormous effort. From brushing your teeth, to fixing your hair, to dressing, we took our time. We teased and giggled. We knew we were getting married, we couldn't wait, and yet there was no rush. We knew that all we had to look forward to was around us now, that this moment was our future. Sometimes you don't get more time, so you take what you can get. We stayed in between your pace and mine. I dressed you slowly, making sure you were perfectly presentable. It took us over an hour. You looked incredibly handsome, smiling broadly. You were radiant. Your mother bought a gorgeous gardenia corsage and pinned it carefully to your chest, telling you just how handsome you were. The fragrance filled the room. It was quarter to ten when Laura knocked on the front door. I was still in my pajamas when she said good morning.

"Honey what are you doing?" She eyed my polar bear pajamas.

"I've been helping my fiancée get ready."

You pointed to me, mouthed to Laura, "That's my fiancée," and smiled.

She snickered at the two of us so playful. “But it’s almost eleven, the wedding is about to start. I think it’s time for YOU to get out of your PJs.”

...

Women have dresses we know we look good in. Our boobs perky, our waist tiny, our butt and legs firm. I’m not vain. I just know I look good in it. My dress is lavender, and against tanned skin, it looks amazing. Stunning. Sexy. It’s my go-to dress, my would-be wedding dress. You’ve seen me in the dress before, at a premiere party we attended. The dress didn’t last a minute once we got home. You instantly peeled it off, carried me to the bedroom, and left it in a pile on the floor.

I rummaged through the closet, knew it was on a hanger somewhere in my sea of clothes. Flipping through hanger after hanger took me some time, but finally I spotted the familiar lavender swatch of fabric. “Ah-ha.” I pulled the dress from the closet and took it off the hanger, shook out its silky fabric and laid it on the bed. I noticed another dress hanging. A dress I bought three years ago at a thrift store. Forgot about the dress completely. It was floor-length cream and lace. The straps were wide linen with lace overlay to the waist. Pearl buttons trailed down the front, to the tied waist. A 1970s summer wedding dress.

I tried on the wedding dress. I slipped it over my shoulders and let it slide down my legs to the floor. I zipped the side, straightened the silk under-slip. I wasn't expecting it to fit flawlessly, but it did. The dress was elegant, fetching. A wedding dress waiting for its day to be adored. It was a beautiful dress. In it I stood up straighter and felt amazing in a garment I'd bought before I even knew when I would wear it.

Considering my tears from our proposal dinner, there was no point putting on makeup. I washed my face, applied lotion, a little blush and lip gloss. I wore stunning ruby earrings my dad had given my mother one wedding anniversary, which she had passed on to me. I combed my hair, twisted back strands into a blue bobby-pin with baby's breath.

"I'm ready," I said to myself in the mirror and then again out loud to the hallway. Twenty minutes and I was ready to get married.

I didn't want to come out of the bathroom and have you see me in my wedding dress. It was bad luck, and we couldn't afford any more bad luck. So I sat on the toilet seat and waited. I was nervous to see you. I was hoping you were nervous, too. I practiced my vows as I heard the doorbell ring and your mother's voice answering. There was a conversation but the door was closed and I couldn't hear the words. Your mother knocked on the bathroom door a moment later, and handed me a gorgeous bouquet of red roses tied together with a luscious white ribbon. A perfect arrangement for a perfect day.

"I'm not sure who they are from, but I think these are for you?" She handed me the roses.

I opened the card.

THIS IS SO I CAN WALK YOU DOWN THE AISLE. I LOVE YOU. DAD.

I was a puddle of emotions sitting on the edge of the toilet cradling roses. I was breaking down, and I wasn't sure how to stop crying. Your mother stood in the bathroom not wanting to leave my side. I gazed up at her and tried to grin. She too was in tears not knowing if she should hold me or walk away. "You look beautiful," she declared as I sniffled and examined my roses. I was a mess. Words got in the way of what I wanted to say to your mother, to tell her I loved her, but only tears came out.

There was another knock on the door and Laura entered. She examined the two of us sobbing, then announced, "I think it's time."

...

Isn't it strange how a simple sentence can change you from the person you were to the person you are? The question you asked was no question at all. "Yes. A hundred times, yes. Of course I will marry you!" I had never known completeness like I knew it being wrapped in your arms the night you asked. My fingertips holding onto the cracks of you. Hugging the very foundation of a house of cards. There came a point, maybe when you said the words, "Marry me," that death stopped being scary. What starting being scary was knowing I would be alone. Going on without you. The fear was a flood that threatened to drown me in tears.

I thought being your wife would feel like water wings keeping me afloat. I know: I jumped into the deep-end of love knowing I would lose it all. I knew I would be alone. I knew the timeline. I was counting the days on my fingers. I knew you were going to die. I knew my heart would break because of it. Yet, no matter how fleeting or tragic, I believed in love. I believed in us. I would marry you freely and happily because that is the lunacy of love. I would make you a proud spouse, because I couldn't make you live.

...

Laura stayed in the bathroom with me. "She is right. You do look absolutely beautiful." She handed me Kleenex hidden beneath her robe. "Okay..." She tucked the loose hairs behind my ear. "Do you have something old, something new, something borrowed, and something blue?"

I had forgotten the rhyme. I'm not even sure what the rhyme is for. I asked Laura what it meant. "I'm not exactly sure, but my idea is that each represents a good-luck token. 'Something old' symbolizes family and the past. 'Something new' means optimism and hope for your new life ahead. 'Something borrowed' reminds the bride that she can depend on her friends and family..."

I went through the list. "Ummm, let's see. I have on my mother's earrings…"

"Family and the past." Laura nodded.

"Something new? Um, my BLUE hairclip!" I clapped my hands delighted.

"Perfect. Now something borrowed?"

I studied my arms and down my dress evaluating each item. "I don't really have anything borrowed."

Laura inspected the room, then her own body. "Ah." Her cheeks grinned as she undid the clasp of a small gold cross necklace that hung at the base of her throat. "I've had this since I was a little girl." She stood behind me, and positioned it around my neck. "There." She said satisfied and lovingly. "Now you're ready."

Your mother re-entered the bathroom, concerned. "What is it?" I asked. She informed us that you were too weak to get out of bed but fighting with your body to get up and sit under the elm tree as planned. She didn't think you should use all of your energy on the act of getting up, but instead for the ceremony itself.

"Is it okay if we have the wedding in your bedroom? I think he's too weak without the pain meds…"

"Tell him if he gets out of bed he's going to be divorced before he's even married." We all giggled and then laughed and then really laughed loud. Laughter didn't belong in the moment, or maybe it did. "If we have the wedding in the backyard or bedroom or on this toilet… I will be wherever he is." We stopped laughing.

even if i am.

...

Yesterday we thought maybe your stepfather could play the cello, or the harpist from the church could come, but time didn't permit luxuries and we never formed a backup plan. When Laura asked if we had a wedding march or if there was a song we'd like to play as I walked down the aisle, I didn't know what to say. I simply shook my head no. Shit, I can't believe WE, we of all people, forgot about a wedding song.

Laura thought for a second, saw my disappointment and my tears and then started. Slow at first, then loud enough for everyone to hear. "Daa na na na, daa na na naaah..." I was instantly laughing mixed with crying and could hear your parents and then you and hospice, maybe Gladys too, singing the wedding march. I walked slowly from the bathroom through the hallway across the living room and into the bedroom. I was holding my dad's hand in the form of red roses. He felt close enough to touch. My mother's whisper in my ear. Gladys was prancing and snorting with all the excitement of singing, and skipped alongside.

We entered the room, I couldn't take my eyes off yours. I'm sorry I was such a puddle, but you were, too. We all were. Your mother, hospice, Laura... Even your stepfather's shirt was wet around the neck. "Good God, we're all a mess," I said as we chuckled, wiping tears with wet sleeves. I couldn't resist leaning in to nestle your nose. Your hand grabbed the back of my head, pulling me closer, not letting go, as Laura began.

"We are gathered on this beautiful afternoon to share in everlasting love..."

As she continued the ceremony you sneaked in little whispers, little cuddles. "You are beautiful. The most beautiful thing I have ever seen. I am the luckiest man in the world." Laura continued the tradition as my tears mixed with yours in between nestling noses. "I hope you know just how much I love you." You spoke in a steady, soft stream of words. "I love you. I love you so much."

I could only get out the words. "I love..."

Laura stopped midway through the ceremony and said, "You know you guys can't kiss yet, right?"

We both snickered. You said, "We haven't, but I want to."

"First, let's get through the vows. Are you ready?" We both nodded. "Do you Anthony Rigby Glass take Chasity Rae..."

You remained so present, so happy. I loved the way you said "I do." I loved the way you smiled when I did.

I knew our marriage would be brief and end in sorrow. I knew the timeline. I knew it well. But, seeing you emotionally naked and fragile in your illness, all I could think of was love. Infinite love—immeasurable love—vast, immense, glorious, fat love, the kind of love you search for your entire life. The kind of love that never dies. The kind of love that surrounds you, fills you, completes you. The kind of love that kills cancer.

Laura later described our matrimony as an extraordinary witness of such love, of amazing courage and personal sacrifice. While stumbling over my vows, my mind prayed to Poppy, "Please don't take him from me. Please don't take him. Take me, instead." I somehow thought with a reverend standing across from me, my prayers would finally be heard. I used her to help me talk to God. Used her to help me save you. Surely God saw how happy we were. That your love was safe with me.

"You may kiss the bride."

...

We should have taken more photographs. Fourteen total. That's all we took. We were too busy hugging and crying, and I think we clapped after your stepfather gave a heartfelt speech on marriage. I only remember because there is a photo of it, of us clapping. There were laughs on lips and teeth, smiles and Kleenex. Gladys sat at your bedside. I love looking through the fourteen photos. Reminding myself of the moments, I can still hear your mother's wonderment when you asked Laura to continue the ceremony.

"I'm ready," you stated to Laura as she nodded in agreement. I took a photograph.

She requested that your mother and stepfather each grab a hand of yours to hold. I stood at the foot of the bed.

She began, "Blessed is the child of light who is pure in heart, for that person shall see God. For as the heavenly

Father has given you, Anthony, his Holy Spirit, and your earthly mother has given you her holy body…" Suddenly I saw your mother's understanding in the way she held your hand securely, in the way she began to weep. Baptism was a sacrament she never did with you as a child, something she regretted, something that meant a great deal to her in her own faith. You knew the significance of the ritual. You knew what the rite meant to her. You needed her to know that you were unhurt and now safe with God. That she did fix you—she saved you because she loved you.

The ceremony was short, effortless and untouched. You never took your eyes off your mother's adoring silent sentiments. She marked a cross on your forehead in holy oil as you closed your eyes receiving the prayer with a euphoric welcome.

"Baptized in the name of the Father and of the Son and of the Holy Spirit."

Amen. I took another photo.

…

My heart felt as if it might break through my bones, rip out of my chest and land in your lap, offering itself to you wholly, thanking you for you. My heart wanted to go with you wherever you went. It wanted to find a home in the pocket of your pink shirt. Become a neighbor to your heart. You could knock on my heart's door and borrow a cup of sugar to make sweet tea. We could sip that tea and discuss our day.

I felt it most when I watched you sleep. I couldn't imagine that you were comfortable, curled up in your wedding clothes, though you appeared to be. Your breath, slow and irregular, told me more than words could. It sounded like there was foam in the back of your throat. I swallowed. I assumed it was the higher dose of pain medication you were now on. I tried to give you a drink, but you were too sleepy to wake. Instead you smiled at something happy, wrapped in dream I would never see. I wished I could crawl into it with you, where hearts beat and pulses rise and hopes are high. I tucked the inch of overgrown hairs behind your ear, noticing the beads of perspiration shining alongside the oiled cross on your forehead. Your hand still a tight fist on your chest. Your wedding ring two sizes too big, in danger of slipping off. You were still grinning, fast asleep clutching your wedding ring hand placed perfectly on your chest to keep it safe.

I snuggled into the twin bed and alongside your warm body. I couldn't resist you a moment more. "Hello, husband," I muttered to the side of your neck.

You reached for my arm to pull me closer. "I just had the most amazing dream."

"You did? What did you dream?"

"I dreamt I married an angel." You held up your fist, still tight, ring still on. I leaned in and brushed your shoulder with my lips, then gently curled up closer, resting my arm across your chest and whispered. "I love you, hubby."

"I love you more, wifey."

...

We invited twelve people to our wedding reception, and twelve came. I thought you could spend some time with Jane, Zach and Jay before the party started. They hadn't seen you in weeks, if not months. I never asked if you wanted a reception—I told you. That's what spouses do.

As guests arrived they congratulated your parents and hugged me hello then asked to see you. We knew most of your friends would be overwhelmed by your appearance. I knew I needed to prepare them.

"I know it's been a while since you've seen Anthony, but there are some things I need to tell you first." I told them that you had lost a bit of weight. When you closed your eyes to sleep, they didn't shut fully. Your skin and eyes were yellow. That today, after the ceremony, you were on oxygen and a stronger dose of pain medication. I told them that you were frail, but absolutely coherent and that you would do your very best to whisper something back.

I woke you from your nap. "Hey, babe, Jane is here to see you."

You smiled the second you saw her. I wanted to give her private time to share with you and tell you everything she needed to say.

She gave you a kiss on the cheek. "Hello."

After a few minutes with Jane, I went to check on the two of you. Your expressions were timid, trying to stay awake. "Jane, can you help us out in the kitchen?"

"Absolutely." She was upset but remained collected.

"Sorry, babe, but you have to share your time. Jay is here now. Would you like to say hi?"

...

I prepped every friend, then left the room, helping in the kitchen, greeting more guests. I would return after a few minutes passed to make sure your energy was holding up, that you were drinking your Ensure, that you didn't need help to go to the bathroom. You were getting worn out, even after the first visit. You and I guessed it was going to be emotional for your friends. You were going to be as hopeful and as cheerful as you could. Yet, I don't think we really factored in how equally emotional it would be for you, or how tiresome. Jay's visit was the most affecting. I prepped him. Left the room, then came back after ten minutes.

When I entered and you mumbled to Jay, "Jaybone, I love you. It's going to be okay." Jay left the room, and you began to cry. "This is harder than I thought it would be."

"I know." I rubbed my nose in your hair. "I know."

"Thank you." You grabbed my arm tightly, not wanting me to leave your side, "Wife."

Bill and Sam entered the room with their new baby girl, Dakota, maybe a couple months old. You held up your fist and said, "I'm a spouse. Maybe I'll be father someday, too." Dakota was the first to giggle. Your eyes lit when you heard her.

I slipped out of the room and eavesdropped on Jane and Jay in the kitchen. "I can't believe Glassanova got married," Jane said. I poured myself a drink and pretended I didn't hear.

I remember telling everyone the story of your proposal, of your parents as waitstaff, and the food. I remember posing for a picture. You weren't in it. We were toasting our wedding day. Your parents and I thought it best to let you rest while we cheered with the other guests. Someone gave a speech—your mother maybe. I just remember fighting back tears, but smiling, a nothing-held-back kind of one. I wanted to crumble now, in front of them. I didn't. Instead, I raised my glass, ate grocery store chocolate cake. Nothing fancy or prepared for the event, a generic chocolate cake with white frosting roses on top. I saved you a bite, one with fudge in the middle. Chocolate cake and ice cream, fat love in a bite.

You stayed in bed as guests filed out begrudgingly, wanted to say goodbye one last time. No one wanted to leave. They would have stayed all night if given the chance.

...

I unpinned your corsage, placed it gently on the nightstand as you looked at me with love. "It should be forever," you told me in barely a whisper, harmonizing over the oxygen filling tubes. "God told me..."

"A—" was all I could voice before the tears came, wetting the words. I could not speak. A simple I love you seemed perfect on our wedding night, yet I couldn't even say your name. Instead I brought my cheek to yours, nestled and kissed your earlobe. Our lashes intertwined as the oxygen tube, soft and cold, nuzzled between. The world stood still in our house, in our bed, in our burrowed expressions. It should be forever, and it was. We lived in our forever with kisses, and tears, and the right-then.

"Promise me you'll be okay when I'm gone," you said as my cheek brushed against your lips.

"I promise," I lied.

...

"I think you should sleep in the room with us tonight," I said to your mother.

"But it's your wedding night."

"I know... I know. It's just..." I paused. I searched for the right words, but none seemed fitting so I just blurted sentences. "Anthony's lived his life fully today. He married his love. He got to see his friends and say goodbye. He got to hear their love for him and share his own. He's the happiest he will ever be. He wants you there. He wants his mother at his bedside tonight. He wants to share his love. Share his peace."

"I'd be honored to share this night with you."

. . .

I remember it well. There was sleep in your eyes. Time stopped moving. Your mother and I took turns watching you sleep throughout the night. One of us would sit at your bedside while the other would try to get some rest. There was one part of the night when you started talking and yelling or arguing to someone else in the room. Someone behind the walls, behind the streets, towns, and states, behind the stars. I couldn't understand what you were saying. I took your hand in mine and pushed the play button on your pain medication. I wet your lips with a mint flavored sponge. Hospice came into the room and Gladys, too. She barked, startling us, seeming really upset. Staring in the same direction you were.

I yelled at her, "Gladys, go lay down!"

She did something strange. She laid at the foot of the doorway to our bedroom, a place she had never rested before, and kept guard. Like she knew someone else was in the room. Maybe I'm crazy. You always said I was a little crazy at times but there was this amazing mystical way of the room. The energy shifted and changed. Goosebumps and hairs standing on end. Someone was there communicating with you and you seemed upset with him.

Hospice put a hand on my shaking shoulder and said, "It's time. Time to hold him. Time to tell him it's okay to go." Your mother and I each held your hand. I rubbed your head because I knew you liked that. I wanted you to know I was close.

"I'm okay, babe. I'll be okay. I love you. I love you so much. I love you. It's okay... You can go now. I love you." Each word destroyed me.

Your mother continued my sentiments. "I'll continue loving you. Thank you for the blessing of being your mother. I am so proud of you. I love you..."

I was numb. Shocked. Stunned. I remember holding your hand and how it grew instantly lifeless. Your soft knuckles under my thumb, the movement of your skin with the brush of my finger, smooth, then wrinkled. The rattling, percolating sounds with each breath. Dreaming and smiling. The smell of baby powder and sweat and mint. Your breath shallow and deep, soft and slow. You opened your eyes to stare off in a corner to cough, to sigh. I rubbed your chest for your comfort, or my own. Your eyes never focused on me.

I said, "Squeeze my hand one last time, babe. Remind me again that you love..."

You clutched our fingers as tight as you could, feeling weak and soft.

Then took your last breath.

...

I wanted to climb on top of you and let the breath of your lungs push me up and down. I wanted to rest my face on your chest and check for signs of life.

"I love your skinny arm." I kissed it. "I love your soft cheeks." I kissed them. "I love your nose." Kissed it. "I love your earlobes. Did I ever tell you, you have the world's softest earlobes? I love your earlobes. I love you." I kissed them. "I love you more," I said, but you were already gone.

I held you there. Your eyes got black and your breath stopped and your body got tight. There are things about death that no one tells you. Things that are gross and descriptive and smell weird. It took me a while to disconnect. I waited for it to sink in, to feel you gone. I wanted a brochure. I wanted to read about what I was supposed to be feeling, or doing. You were lying in front of me—I could touch you, feel you, but you were no longer you. Just a body ridden with cancer.

I didn't move for hours, or maybe it was only minutes. Time does strange things when you love a person with cancer.

Hospice came in, starting singing a hymn and doing what hospice does, the angels of death, loving the soul and honoring the beauty of death. She undressed you slowly, bathed you one last time, leaving the cross on your forehead. Singing throughout her movements. You were naked. Peaceful. Transcending the physical world as she closed your eyes and crossed your hands over your chest. I know I wanted to cry but I couldn't. I didn't. I only watched you lie there.

My breathing became shallow. The two sides of my brain stopped talking to each other. I'm not sure I even had a brain at this point. My responses were distant and glossed-over, as in a movie where everything around the actor is motion but their body is still. A freeze frame. I felt disconnected and unsafe. I had this strong urge to get drunk or self-medicate. Waves of overwhelming numbness paralyzed my ability to cope or even stand up. I was caught in the moment, taking a picture of a worrisome scene.

Your mother turned on classical music. I sat and watched your body as a solo violin started the concerto. Waiting for you to take another breath, to tell your mother to turn the music down. A fly landed on your eyelashes, making his way to your eye. I waved my hands across your face to startle him. "Shoo fly." This is what I probably said, or maybe I didn't say anything at all. The increased volume and richer sound of the music had me standing over your body. Not wanting to touch you, but protecting you from a housefly. Everything slowed down. The image of you blurred and the voices in the distance faded. All I heard was the buzzing. Buzzing mixed with the orchestral melody.

The fly landed on my chest. I glanced down, not even realizing until then that I was still wearing my wedding dress.

chapter fifty-one

a classical station

Two men from the morgue came. They wore navy blue suits. They entered the house with a stretcher and a green body bag. Gladys growled, trying to bite the metal wheels along the hardwood. She knew this machinery was here to take you and she did not approve. I had to carry her outside as the men came to do what they were paid to do; pick up and remove a body in a bag. A body. You were no longer a name or a personality or even a sex. You were a body.

"Miss, you'll need to remove any valuables from the body first."

I was confused—you weren't wearing anything. You were naked.

"You need to remove his wedding ring," your mother said.

You still had a fist. I worked the band off your finger, and started crying as they lifted your body. Knowing this would be the last time I would see you.

. . .

I called my father. He said he would be on the next flight, and he was.

I called my mother. She cried, saying the word sorry over and over.

. . .

I didn't know who to call next, or what to do, or the protocol. I didn't know where to begin. I called the sweetest voice I knew; I called Julie. I asked her if she could call Jay first. He would've been the first person I called if I had the strength.

"I'll call as soon as we hang up."

"Thank you, Jules."

"Is it okay if I come later tonight to check in..."

"Yes. I'd like that."

"Chas, I'm so sorry."

"Me too." I could hear her whimper as we said goodbye.

I called Kaethy at the office next and left a message.

. . .

All of a sudden the house was active. I didn't realize just how many people and medical supplies were in each room. I was thankful your stepfather was there; he did all the planning and paperwork and logistics. I just said yes or no to decisions, signed things, wrote checks. He made funeral plans and meal plans and flight plans and crematory plans. He did everything. Your mother and I just sat on the couch staring at an empty television, trying to comprehend the events around us.

...

Babe, can we talk? I need to tell you something. I need you to know that I am sorry. I'm sorry I pushed you to see your friends, pushed you too hard during the ceremony. Why did I agree to stopping the pain medication? I knew you were exhausted after the wedding. I should have cancelled the reception and planned it for another day. I think it was too much. I pushed you too hard. I shouldn't have. I regret being selfish. Maybe you would've stayed with me for a few more days, if only I hadn't pushed you so hard. It's my fault, and baby, I'm sorry. I thought we had weeks left. I didn't know what to do.

...

"Zach?"

"Hiii..."

"He's gone."

"Fuck. I know, I talked to Julie."

"He's gone Zach and..."

"I'm here."

"I don't know what to do."

"I'm here if you need anything." Pause. "Chas?"

"I don't know what to do..."

"You keep loving him, that's what you do."

"But what if I forget..."

"You won't, because he wouldn't let you."

...

I didn't know what to do. I know I was loved but, for some reason I was caught up in how fast your disease came and how short our time was. I was caught up and angry at your prognosis, and how ineffective your treatments were. I was so caught up in the idea that I pushed you too hard, that I forgot—I forgot you loved me.

I know. It's foolish. I wished you were there so I could tell you all the things I forgot to say or kiss the parts of your body I missed, like the backs of your knees. Why didn't I kiss them? I wish you were here now. I'd kiss the shit out of your knees.

...

I grabbed the book you made me for Christmas, the book of all the e-mails we sent. I turned to July 27th, exactly a year ago.

Remind me I am loved. Tell me what to do.

chapter fifty-two

i couldn't attach the song i wanted to send with this

"We believe that Anthony is at peace. We saw that in his last days he achieved his solitude, even in the presence of weakness, discomfort, and impending death. We remember joyful smiles, tender words, and deep affection to Chas and those around him, even at the very end. The cancer defeated his body, but nothing defeated his spirit."

Laura, our reverend, continued the service as I looked around at all the faces. Some I knew, some I didn't. Some wept, others stared blankly ahead. I wander back and forth from face to face, not making eye contact. I felt the sadness roll into crashing doubts of everything in my life. I had no ability to make meaning in the suits and blazers and high heels. I want it to be over. Get out of this fitted black dress and back into my pajamas.

How could you leave me here, babe, listening to your brother reading a eulogy, actually telling the church that you "had skills with women."

"He had mastered and understood women almost a decade ahead of his time."

I was laughing, but acting as if I were in tears. I looked around the church. I saw Jay, a familiar face; he too was laughing but I thought it might be a cover-up for his tears. This gave me the giggles. Do wives giggle at their husband's funeral? My dad sat to my left. Crying. I'd never seen my dad cry before. Funny to think that you were the one making him cry, babe. He was so quiet. His tears go almost unnoticed. He was gazing at the photo of you at the head of the church.

"It's okay, Dad." He looks up at me. "I'm okay." I held his clammy hand for comfort. He looked back up at the photo. It was the one of you visiting your grandmother. You have this big toothy smile as your grandmother takes the photo.

My dad caught his breath. "I'm meeting your husband for the first time."

I was senseless. You never met my dad. I forgot.

Jay walked up to the podium. He looked sad and I bet that he wouldn't get through the first sentence. "You, Anthony, were so kind to this world." Jay stood strong and steady, grabbing my attention. "In a world that is full of selfishness and indifference, a small gaze of compassion from your strong, kind eyes would soften the hearts of so many who were calloused and jaded." Jay sounded like a public speaker, a politician. "Anthony has always been my rock that I cling to in times of despair and sadness, and I was lucky enough to spend a little bit of time with him on his last day, and as he lay there taking some of his last breaths, he could see me trying to hold back the tears, he could sense my fear and sadness. In an effort to console ME, he turned his head, held my hand so tight, gazed at me with those selfless, kind eyes, and in such a soft, sweet, tired voice whispered, 'Its gonna be okay.' And it IS gonna be okay because you, Anthony, with your unconditional friendship, love, and happiness, you have set an example for us all. So go, my friend, go in peace knowing that you are loved, and keep with you the happiness that you have found in YOUR true love, and know that one day, together, we will rejoice in that again." But Jay was sobbing by the end. "You will always be my rock. I love you, Anthony." I stand to give Jay a hug. I turned to your mother, and she placed her hand on my shoulder with her wet handkerchief. Her voice is dry and shaky. "That was beautiful." We look at the floor and we don't speak. We hold hands and we breathe and we think.

Zach was now standing at the podium reading, "You're probably sitting there wondering why I've worn a pink shirt to Anthony's memorial service, so let me just put the rumor to rest that I have shockingly bad taste." Zach had the church laughing. "I was talking with friends the day Anthony passed and it was noted that I had a touch of pink on my shirt. I mused that I wasn't willing to go much further into pink-wearing territory. The right opportunity to wear pink hadn't quite presented itself yet. Maybe five hours later, Chas was recounting the wedding in all its beautiful details. As was always the case, Anthony had taken great care in making sure his clothes were all dialed in. He had decided to wear a pink shirt, because he 'didn't want to wear white.' Well, I for one took that as a sign. Antone, always a guru of fashion, wasn't going to let me neglect such a stylish section of the color palette. So, Tony, this one's for you..."

I was smiling at Zach, so thankful that he was reading and we were laughing and my dad was no longer crying. Zach had this way of making me forget things like the past or the future or the laundry I left in the washer. I always got caught up in listening to his stories, using words like level-headed and cool. I know that I've met new people, made new friends, but I am starting to think Zach was heaven-sent. He understood us, shared in our joys and pains. He was a part of our story.

"As Anthony and Chas," Zach resumed, " started to date, I found myself witnessing the genesis of an amazing relationship. Chas and I had become friends after working on a terrible DVD project a few months back. Wouldn't it just figure that my two closest friends at work would fall in love. Anticipating the future, I thought about getting the words 'third wheel' tattooed on my arm.

"I wish you all could know how sweet and beautiful their courtship was. I found myself taking notes on the way they treated each other. If I were to use just half of the things Anthony did, I could write a best-selling how-to book on making a girl fall head over heels. I watched them operate and I thought, that is what love is. That's what I want for myself one day."

Each eulogy was a mirror of the reader. Your parents and I agreed on who would deliver them. We asked each person individually. Each accepted it as a great honor. Every eulogy wanted to make you proud: Jay, Zach, a childhood friend, your brother, and I. We listened to the stories and imagined what your life was all about. We learned. We remembered. We wanted someone to tell us that your life meant something, that all of us meant something. Each eulogy gave us the chance to focus on the you we all loved, the whole you: your strengths, your joys, challenges and achievements.

"I have tried more than once to prepare myself for this day," Zach continued. "I have been overcome with sadness the last few months, and I didn't think I would know how to handle this. But I find myself thinking now that I'll always have Anthony with me, because I am always thinking, 'What would he do here, or what would he say?' I can hear him telling me to pump the brakes when I'm doing something dumb. I can hear him telling me to rally when I'm moping around. When something goes wrong, I can hear his one-word sympathy, suck, that somehow means so much. And as I look around the room, every one of your faces reminds me of him. I've been so scared of what life would be like without him, but I realize now that he's always with me, and it makes me feel like I can one day be the man, friend, and husband that he was."

It was a blur of words, a daze of sentiments. I was mixed up with emotions, feeling human and in need of God. I looked inside myself trying to find a way to trust God again. Collecting my sadness, I closed my eyes. I was mad at God for leaving me behind. Yet I prayed anyway and prayed honestly. *Poppy, give me strength.* I took a deep breath. Amen. Then shuffled my way to the front of the church.

"Most of you know Anthony was an amazing writer. He was a great kisser too, but that's not what I'm here to tell you about." The church giggled. "I'm going to read an e-mail he wrote me at a time in my life when I needed answers. He was such an amazing writer. His words could save you. His words could wrap themselves around you and protect you. You could fall in love with his words. I did. Okay, maybe it helped he was a good kisser..." The church giggled again. "I wanted to share with you an e-mail he wrote me exactly a year ago from the day he passed. I went to his e-mails looking for signs and reassurance, to know that I would be all right. To look for an answer in all of this. I'm sorry if I choke on his words..." I turn to Laura, "And I am sorry I am about to swear in church." I can hear Jay laugh, or cry.

From: le_samurai@yahoo.com
To: chasityrae@gmail.com
Sent: Wednesday, July 27, 10:22 a.m.
Subject: i couldn't attach the song i wanted to send with this...

and that sucks because it was perfect

i couldn't attach the song i wanted to send with this

i am scared
of being scared...
and so,
i am not.

even if i am.

for too much of my life,
at the worst times, some random times
and inevitably embarrassing times,
my hands have shaken...

despite me.
my efforts to focus.
calm.
steady...

FUCK!

and it is a sad betrayal
when your body gives up your mind,
shows that which you would conceal,
that which you cannot...

but something good
has come out of it...

even if i am.

and that is,
i know i still must act.
must push through it,
must do whatever it is.

fear is familiar.
and so,
when it comes
i know what to do.

"my fear is my only courage
so i have to push on through..."
—bob marley

i know...
i can't believe i just quoted bob marley either,
but it came to mind,
and even if i sound like
a college freshman...
it helps the point.

despite your efforts
to illustrate the contrary,
i don't think you are fearful.

i think you are bold.
and i think you are beautiful.
i think you are bold and beautiful.

i couldn't attach the song i wanted to send with this

(oh christ, i'm losing it...)

but there is something inside of you,
something i have seen:
a strength. steadiness. courage.

as opaque as you are.
it is easy to see.

perhaps you are scared now,
frozen by the fear you feel
because you don't know
how to handle it...

fear is not familiar for you.

we are defined by
who we are in crisis...
you are overwhelmed.

so quit your fucking whining
and do something about it.

something amazing.
because that is who you are.
that is what i see.

chapter fifty-three

track 3

Saturday, September 15

I wonder if I am supposed to cry this much, because it seems like that's all I do. I cry when I'm in the shower, wake up, before bed, in the car, go for a walk, when I read a book, get dressed, breathe. I cry.

I try to put on this believable game face with friends and family. I never cry in front of them. Instead I give animated smiles and positive status reports to my grieving process. Everyone usually seems pleased with my response, and compliments me on my strength. I've come up with generic answers to favored questions like, "How are things?" "How's work?" "You doing okaaay?" I give them stock replies because my honest answers would cause most people to worry. If okay means I need sleeping pills to rest at night, or I've lost ten pounds in two months, or I eat bags of popcorn for dinner because I don't want to cook for only one—then yes, I'm doing fine.

Sunday, November 25

I have this reoccurring dream. I carry around your head. No body, no shoulders even. Disgusting, I know. But I tell people "it is all I have left and I am afraid to let it go." I carry it around. Look at your sweet face. Change the bandage on your cheek. Kiss your forehead and nuzzle your face, like we use to do, like Eskimos. Your lips form a half moon and smile back, as I place your sleeping head back into my bag. Everywhere I go. You are with me.

I'm careless in the few memories I have left of you. I'm composing settings all my own while creating scenarios of untruths. "Remember that time we traveled to Bali for our wedding anniversary?" Developing a mind's snapshot to frame rather than repetitiously filing memories true. I've lost our memories to my desire of wanting you here. I'm sorry. But you left me with so few. I don't have thirty years like your mother, or numerous good times like friends. I barely have a year. I'm afraid a single memory might slip through the cracks of my fingers, not unlike holding water. No matter how tight I squeeze my fingers, I'm afraid I might lose you. I have so little to grasp.

As a result I've continued my elliptical march of filing memories to a place I won't forget, squeezing my hands so tight not to lose you. I place your sleeping head in my bag. Everywhere I go. You are with me.

Thursday, February 14

resembling that of a phantom limb,
an element of me no longer connected.
today grief feels like an amputation.

like an absent piece of self;
an absent piece of something whole,
something familiar.
half of a whole.

I am learning to take my first steps with artificial legs,
learning to embrace with my torso, and not both arms.
is it possible to become an amputee of an emotion?
such as love?
a hole so vast in your chest, breathing becomes difficult.

how do you pray for a missing piece
that is a part of your own heart?

still, there is no denying that in some sense I do, feel better.
my phantom love has now become my prosthetic sorrow.

careers are on the horizon.
a healthy Gladys skipping alongside.
my friends near.
my family close.
as I learn to take first steps, as half of a whole.
and finding some joy in between.

...

Anthony, I've been writing this story, wonderfully wondering what I should include and disclose. It's hard to not want to skip ahead, past the daily doses of disease and grieving journal entries and discontent and get to the good days. There are good days but there sure were a ton of bad ones. The months I'd hoped to spend with you were hijacked by malignancies—they told us maybe a year, months, certainly not days. When you asked me if I'd be okay without you, I lied. I mean I did, and I didn't. That first year without you, I felt lost, fending for myself in a daunting landscape of being alone. This unquenchable emptiness eating away at my soul, my stomach, my insides. Trying to understand what the word grief meant. I asked myself all too often, "Now what?" I was faced with the scalding reality of being on this side of life without you. I was afraid that if I let go of my sorrow and put out the fire in my heart, I would lose you.

It was the little things that wrecked me, like loading the dishwasher without you, or strolling down every aisle in the supermarket, placing my toothbrush in the slot next to yours. I was learning to take first steps like a child. Learning to walk again. Learning what to do with your tools in the garage and the Cruiser and socks. I still have them, your socks. I didn't know what to do with them. There needs to be a pamphlet for that. On what to do with socks and toothbrushes after someone dies. I started wearing them and your flannels too, sometimes even your deodorant. You felt closer when I did. Sometimes I still wear them.

...

I used to be sad when I thought about this time, that first year alone. What I didn't realize was that it would be filled with people and prayers and lasagna and homemade soups and daisies and sunflowers and paperwork. After the funeral the house filled with people, doing activities. I was never lonely. I had support buzzing around me, helping me, holding me up whenever I wobbled. Gladys had a dozen aunts and uncles to play ball with, to love. Jay even fed her table scraps when I wasn't looking.

An outside friend labeled our home "Camp Mourn." I didn't mind. I was proud of the camaraderie, to be surrounded by such warmth. Julie cooked a turkey that first Christmas. My first birthday York lit the candles on my cake. On Valentine's Day, Jane and I went traveling. On our wedding anniversary, Jay and I ate the frozen chocolate cake from our wedding day and shared stories of you. The cake was disgusting. I'm still not sure why it's tradition to keep frozen cake until the first anniversary. The year of your death we all went for a bike ride to the beach and toasted you with champagne exactly like we did when we spread your ashes. (Remind me to tell you that story.) In August I went to Maine and visited your family.

All the holidays, time markers, days without you, Camp Mourn was there. Always in love, some days in despair, but it was all the same. I certainly wouldn't be where I am today without them. Without that first year and their comfort. Those twelve friends who came to our reception were my wedding gift, my honeymoon, my happily-ever-after. Whenever I miss you, I call them. You live in their stories, in their smiles, in the ways they love, and ways they laugh. Without you I can't imagine anymore.

...

It's been five years since you left. It took me five years to write these pages. Every day is a new piece of my learning. A lot has happened in five years. This entire journey has drawn me into a labyrinth of feelings. I have been able to discover so many aspects of myself, once buried and lost. I no longer believe in words like forever. All that I have is here and now, and that is enough. You taught me that. You taught me that love is the language, the laugh lines, the spaces between the words written and jokes told and stories shared and beers drunk. Love is what living is for. You taught me that sometimes love is something you can't let go of. And sometimes love is something you'd do anything to forget. And sometimes, we learn something about love that changes everything we know about ourselves.

There is so much more I need to tell you. So many more stories—OHMYGOD, York and Julie are MARRIED! Ten years together and they had a secret ceremony, only the two of them. We're still awaiting a rowdy reception. Maybe they'll have one in Portland. They live there now.

Oooh, and you'll never guess who I'm living with these days: Jay. I know, crazy right? He moved into the house shortly after you left to help me stay grounded. "I would love to move in with you and Anthony if you'll let me." Jay is a saint. In all his distance from you and your disease, he helped me a great deal that first year. Listening, not questioning or pushing me along in my grieving. We talked openly about you, both missing you terribly. You'd be proud of him. I know—you're proud of him already. He fixed up the Cruiser. She looks amazing with new fabric and tires and transmission and he even replaced the cracked dashboard.

Gladys still sits in the passenger seat panting with her face out the window, lips flapping in the wind. She is a funny dog. She's getting old now, twelve this year. Not sure how much time she has left, but I think she's ready. She'll be so excited to see you.

Um, let's see—Zach continues his travels. I think he's somewhere in Europe now, Bulgaria maybe, trying to find his sense of purpose. I think he's going to end his two-year journey in India. I'll be curious to see if he still has his heart intact or if he's given it away completely.

As for Jane, you were right, she is an amazing friend, and the perfect travel companion. Spain was our first destination. I even brought along your journal from your trip with Jay. I read about your rowdy Spain travels and the girl and the drinks and the cities. I filled the back pages of the journal with my own adventures.

You've missed such good music the last couple of years, like Bon Iver and Greg Laswell and Passion Pit and Angus and Julia Stone and the Avett Brothers. I swear, some of the songs were meant for you and me. I like to think you're writing songs in heaven and sending them to me. I am certain you wrote track three on York's latest mix. I don't even know who sings it or the band. All I know is that it is perfect. Thank you.

...

I am doing well. I'm now in a place where there is no more confusion over why you left or why God took you from me. People have told me time heals all wounds. I disagree. Time gives you space and distance and understanding. There is still a scar, an eternal ache, but there is also a bandage of acceptance. I'm in a place where there is only peace and joy and perfect love and gratitude. And I thank God for those things again. I was mad at Him that first year, maybe even the second and third. He was distant and remote and I felt completely abandoned. But I trust in Him again. I told God the truth.

I told him I missed you and every time I thought the words, "miss you," I cried. I'm not sure if that feeling will ever go away. I told Him that. The more I talked to Him, the more I cried, feeling every emotion I had collected along the way. I cried through every stage of grief and then back around again. Round and round. I'm not numb anymore. I am living, breathing, existing at my most raw. I am human and God is always right there. Right where I need Him to be. In my heart. In my love. In my you.

I have held on to a number of voicemail messages in my phone. I listen to them when I need a smile or reminder or something as simple as a voice. Today I erased a bunch of them, leaving me with two left. One is from you. *I miss you, call me.*

The other one is from someone you haven't met. I think you'd like him, though. He reminds me of you in the way he can get me to laugh loud and sudden and squirt beer out of my nose. He feels like Minnesota in the winter of freshly chopped wood and hot cocoa. I feel lighter when he is around. And he makes excellent coffee. That has to count for something. No?

Like I said, a lot has happened in these five years. I've somehow made my way out of Los Angeles, out of the discontent, and headed east. Martha's Vineyard is home these days and I can't imagine a more ideal place from which to write to you today. It's summer, it's July, and I'm thinking of celebrating our wedding anniversary by sipping a Blue Moon on the dock of Menemsha, eating lobster with my friend Jessica. Don't worry, I'll get on a bike, too. I promise.

It feels like you're near. Just beyond my reach. I like that feeling. Anyway, I should get back to coffee and listening to my friend chatter more about experiencing love, instead of trying to figure it all out. Maybe we can talk more tomorrow? I'll continue the story from where we left off and tell you about our infamous bike ride the night we spread your ashes on Venice Beach. Today, I just wanted you to hear our love story again and know I wrote these words for you and no one else.

I miss you. It still makes me cry.

acknowledgments

Simply acknowledging each person listed below isn't nearly enough gratitude.

I've considered getting "I ♥ York" tattooed on my butt, for I could never thank Royal York Funston enough. He believed in this story long before I did. His audio interviews are proof that his heart is pure gold, even if he can be a complete pain in the ass sometimes. To a fantastic artist and friend, I honestly couldn't have done this without your help, York. Thank you.

When I borrowed $3000 from my dad and left all my belongings in my mother's garage, telling my parents I'm moving to Martha's Vineyard to write a book—their love and continued support were amazing to me.

To Gladys my dog, thank you for showing me absolute affection—and for growing old, even with cancer.

To my in-laws, I want you to know how much you mean to me now, and how much you meant to me then. Without your kindheartedness, I wouldn't be smiling as bright as I am today.

Much gratitude to my editor, Sarah Cypher, for reminding me of the strength of perspective.

To the early readers: Jaclyn Thomas, Ann Peterson, Carin Zakes, Catherine Mayhew, Jessica Soleil, Julie Ragland and the remarkable writing group on Martha's Vineyard—thank you for listening with open arms, ears and hearts.

To a loving support group on Martha's Vineyard. I know now, I am not alone in this journey.

To Tim and Kaethy, thank you for adopting me into your family.

A huge, "fat" love-filled thank you to the angels that fit into the title "Camp Mourn."

To Zach, for being the perfect third wheel.

To Jay, thank you for honoring that first year, and for loving Glencoe as much as we did.

To Jane, thank you for helping me stand on my own two feet again.

To every person mentioned within this story, and those I've missed. I am so very proud to have you as a part of our story.

I'm struck by how the grace of God works in my life—Thank you, Grant, for meeting me for coffee and sharing your cancer experience.

Anthony, I hope I've told our story truthfully and lovingly… and babe, I miss you.

www.ingramcontent.com/pod-product-compliance
Lightning Source LLC
Chambersburg PA
CBHW070757280326
41934CB00012B/2958